Death Interrupted

Death Interrupted

The Walrus Books

The Walrus sparks essential Canadian conversation by publishing high-quality, fact-based journalism and producing ideas-focused events across the country. The Walrus Books, a partnership between The Walrus, House of Anansi Press, and the Chawkers Foundation Writers Project, supports the creation of Canadian nonfiction books of national interest.

thewalrus.ca/books

Death
Interrupted

HOW MODERN MEDICINE
IS COMPLICATING THE WAY WE DIE

Blair Bigham, MD

ANANSI

Published in Canada in 2022 and the USA in 2022 by House of Anansi Press Inc.
www.houseofanansi.com

House of Anansi Press is committed to protecting our natural environment.
This book is made of material from well-managed FSC®-certified forests,
recycled materials, and other controlled sources.

House of Anansi Press is a Global Certified Accessible™ (GCA by Benetech)
publisher. The ebook version of this book meets stringent accessibility standards
and is available to students and readers with print disabilities.

26 25 24 23 22   1 2 3 4 5

Library and Archives Canada Cataloguing in Publication

Title: Death interrupted : how modern medicine is complicating the way we die /
Blair Bigham.
Names: Bigham, Blair, author.
Identifiers: Canadiana (print) 20220203571 | Canadiana (ebook) 20220203601 |
ISBN 9781487008543
(softcover) | ISBN 9781487008550 (EPUB)
Subjects: LCSH: Terminal care. | LCSH: Death. | LCSH: Medicine.
Classification: LCC R726.8 .B54 2022 | DDC 362.17/5—dc23

Book design: Alysia Shewchuk

*House of Anansi Press respectfully acknowledges that the land on which we operate is the
Traditional Territory of many Nations, including the Anishinabeg, the Wendat, and the
Haudenosaunee. It is also the Treaty Lands of the Mississaugas of the Credit.*

 Canada Council
for the Arts

Conseil des Arts
du Canada

 ONTARIO ARTS COUNCIL
CONSEIL DES ARTS DE L'ONTARIO
an Ontario government agency
un organisme du gouvernement de l'Ontario

With the participation of the Government of Canada
Avec la participation du gouvernement du Canada
 Canadä

*We acknowledge for their financial support of our publishing program the Canada Council
for the Arts, the Ontario Arts Council, and the Government of Canada.*

Printed and bound in Canada

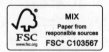

For those who let me into their lives
when everything is crashing down around them

CONTENTS

Introduction

"WHAT ABOUT THIS ONE?" Rakesh hollered at me from across the auditorium-turned-emergency room. He was pointing at a stretcher two paramedics were rolling past him.

"She's dead-dead," I yelled back, before returning to triaging the tidal wave of medical students made up with smoke-streaked faces, red-dyed corn syrup blood, and papier mâché burns.

We were about thirty minutes into a disaster simulation in my medical residency at McMaster University, a test of our hospital's emergency department—and of us as senior residents—to handle an unexpected influx of injured patients. The script was predictable: a nearby soccer stadium had been attacked with improvised explosives, and concerns about chemical weapons were being reported by various sources.

Judges in black T-shirts hovered around with

clipboards, detailing our actions for the debriefing that would follow. Over one hundred patients in one hundred minutes had to be sorted and attended to, and it was my job to assign one of four priorities to each of them and place an index-card-sized triage tag around their necks with a colour to indicate my decision.

· Green was good: it meant they could walk and talk and sit in a chair for hours while we tended to the sickest patients. Yellow was pretty much okay too: they could wait but had the potential to deteriorate. Red was bad: they had injuries like bleeding arteries and collapsed lungs, and required immediate treatment to save their lives. And blue was the worst: they were dead. In the old days, those tags used to be black, and the phrase "black tagged" had become synonymous with "dead." That was why we'd changed the colour to blue — so as not to freak anyone out by slapping a black tag on their friend.

Here's the thing, though. The criteria for a blue tag in a mass casualty situation isn't what you'd think. It doesn't mean you're dead, though you might be. Blue technically stands for expectant — meaning that even if we treated you, you'd still likely die. The tricky part for me, as the triage officer, was that the odds of someone dying was tied to the availability of doctors, nurses, ventilators, surgeons, blood, chest drains, CT scanners, and all the other things that make a hospital tick. If resources were in good supply, the patient was a red — and a trauma team would do everything possible to save their life. But if someone was a blue, they were off to the morgue.

It was up to Rakesh and me, randomly assigned to the two most critical roles in the exercise, to save as many lives as we could. We were both fifth-year residents, and when we weren't training together in the hospital, we often hung out at Synonym or at Truth, two indie coffee shops on gentrified James Street, where we basically camped out for entire days to study or gossip with a constant stream of overpriced caffeine.

If you didn't know him any better, you'd think Rakesh wasn't that interested in being a doctor, but he's just a super mellow guy, which is one of the reasons he became my best friend in residency. So it gave me some amusement to see him amped up during the simulation, yelling at me from the mock trauma bay he was assigned to. It was a sign the simulation was working: we were feeling the heat in the disaster we'd been thrown into by the simulation team.

Rakesh had just opened up a space for another critical patient when he asked me about the body being wheeled past on the stretcher. I'd given her a blue tag. To the many observers, it would appear that he was asking if she was dead. But I knew he really wanted me to say *how* dead I thought she was, whether she was worth the precious resources he was allocating. And not for the first time in my career, I declared the odds to be zero. She was "dead-dead," I told him.

When the phrase came out of my mouth, I took a pause. It wasn't so much an intellectual moment, because there was no time for those. In the chaos of the emergency room, instinct and gut decisions reign. It was more an acknowledgement that "alive" and "dead" aren't black and white. It's not binary, at least not anymore. And for doctors like me, that presents a dilemma of enormous magnitude.

TREATING DEAD PEOPLE IS just part of the job when you're a paramedic or an emergency room nurse or an intensive care doctor. Restoring a heartbeat requires nothing more than solving a physiological riddle. Life requires very little for it to chug along: oxygen, glucose, and heat are the only ingredients needed for the power plants in your cells. As long as you can get those three ingredients from the environment into your body, and circulate them to your nose and toes and everything in between, you can be kept going.

You might hope scientists and doctors could see life and death in a black and white way—a binary construct with clear definitions. I certainly did in my life as a paramedic, where the calls I responded to with lights and sirens blaring had clear-cut stakes: there were those who could be saved, and there were those who proved to be beyond chest compressions, epinephrine, and blood transfusions, who couldn't be saved, no matter our desire or skill or brilliance. The dead-dead.

But as I transitioned from the field to the emergency room and then the intensive care unit, I began to lose clarity around diagnosing death. The line became blurry. And sometimes I didn't really know if a patient was dead or not. That's a problem for a physician. So I decided to write this book to help myself. As I explored a contemporary definition of death, I realized this book might help you too. Because like it or not, everyone you know will die. You will die. I will die. And it's time we stop pretending that isn't the case.

THIS BOOK ISN'T ABOUT terrorist attacks or pandemics, the times when there isn't enough medicine to go around and, like Rakesh and me, we have to prioritize precious resources to those most likely to live. It's about the day-to-day struggle caused by *too much* medicine — the new grey zone caused by the ever-expanding suite of technological and pharmaceutical choices available to doctors that delay a person from being dead-dead but might do little to restore life.

This book is about a place worse than death. A place where doctors despair at the hope families cling to as we poke and prod the patient, pandering to our own egos, afraid to acknowledge that we have failed in our role as life-savers. It is about the space between alive and dead, a space I hope never to occupy personally but one I am guilty of filling, over and over again, with others I'm tasked to care for.

PART I

When Is Dead...Dead?

CHAPTER 1

Policy 4.4

IT ALL STARTED IN the bow of a canoe. I couldn't tell you the when, exactly, since I was just eight weeks old, but in northern Ontario we canoe only three months of the year, when the long summer days make the experience enjoyable. My parents were traversing Crab Lake, which, contrary to its name, has no crabs in it, and the splashes dripping from the blades of their wooden paddles were hitting my face—something I strangely didn't mind, they tell me, and a hint of what was to come. A few hours later, in the middle of a black, quiet lake, my dad took me for a swim. I took to water like a fish. When I was old enough, swimming lessons became the weekly event to look forward to. When it was time to head to Buckler Aquatics, a private pool in an industrial area near the train tracks, I would happily abandon friends, toys, and *Thomas the Tank Engine* on TV.

When I outgrew *Thomas the Tank Engine*, I became obsessed with dramas like ER and *Baywatch*. These were shows in which heroes would rush to perform mouth-to-mouth, or CPR, or defibrillation or emergency surgery, saving lives while looking damn good doing it. According to a study of TV resuscitations, survival rates on television dramas are far higher than in the real world. But I was hooked on a fictional world where lives could easily be saved.

I continued my swimming, earning Bronze Medallion and Bronze Cross awards, which qualified me to join the National Lifeguard service. I timed my lifeguard examination to corne just after my sixteenth birthday, the earliest I could qualify. That summer, I began working at swimming pools at apartment complexes, a boring gig that bore no resemblance to the action-packed episodes of *Baywatch* that had glued me to the television screen.

But at the birthday party of a fellow lifeguard, I was introduced to a couple of paramedics, and this eventually led me to chase in their footsteps. I enrolled in a paramedic program at a college just down the road from where I lived, and by 2006, a week after turning twenty-one, I was a full-time paramedic, proudly suiting up in reflective pants and collared shirts to drive, lights and sirens blaring, from call to call, saving lives and looking, in my own mind at least, like one of my old heroes on TV.

In my work as a paramedic, I pronounced dozens of people dead. It was, at the time, a relatively easy decision to make. The Ministry of Health in Ontario, where I served on ambulances and helicopters for a decade, had a list of things that qualified someone as being "obviously dead." It's the type of list paramedic trainees have to recite for exams and was colloquially known as Policy 4.4.

It included things that didn't really need to be spelled out in a list, like decapitation, rigor mortis, gross charring of a burned body, and obvious decay, which is a far more common thing for a paramedic to find than you might think. In some memorable cases, I pronounced people dead as soon as I stepped off the elevator; the stench coming from their apartment was unmistakable, and the superintendent of the apartment building always knew just as well as I did what we would find on the other side of the occupant's door.

I suppose that would make all the other deaths not obvious, at least if we apply the sterile language of Policy 4.4. But it wouldn't take me long to make the decision. Pulseless, breathless, lifeless. We would perform an assessment, apply a heart monitor, but it was mostly perfunctory. Dead people have a look. As a paramedic, I knew it well.

When death was clear, my work was done. There were no lights and sirens, no hustle, no TV-drama moments. With a look at my watch and a nod to my team, a life was determined to be over. Out came the shrouding white bedsheet (actually, they were a halfway between salmon-pink and faded orange), and I would head out of the room to shatter the life of a stranger.

"I'm sorry to tell you this, but she's dead."

YET SOMETIMES DEATH WAS less clear. There would be no obvious criteria—the look of death had yet to set in—and my mind would race to determine what I could do to pull a person back from the cliff edge. Those were the times adrenalin junkies like me trained for, like an airplane pilot in a simulator when both engines fail. We had a term for patients like this: we'd say they were circling the drain, and we knew that look well too. We'd initiate a choreographed attack on death, two paramedics almost silently executing a series of steps drilled into our minds such that they were as automatic as blinking.

We'd pound hard and fast on the rib cage to eject blood out of the heart. We'd place a breathing tube into the trachea and attach an oxygen-filled bag to it, squeezing air into the lungs like bellows blowing into a fireplace. We would slip a cannula into an arm vein to inject adrenalin directly into the blood so it could reach the heart expeditiously. And, if the stars aligned and we could detect electrical activity in myocytes of the heart, we would defibrillate with an electrical jolt of 200 joules. *Zap.*

Zap. Zap. Zap. My record is thirteen defibrillations on a single patient, far beyond the protocol's three-shock requirement. On scene in a kitchen, then in the driveway, then all the way to the hospital. That time, teams of firefighters rotated through the exhausting chest compressions, keeping blood flowing to the oxygen-sensitive brain, while another paramedic squeezed a ventilation bag. We used our knees and elbows to brace ourselves, sprawled out like spiders for stability, as the rig swung around corners and bounced down city streets, lurching us from side to side.

Zap. Zap. Zap.

We screeched up to the garage door adorned with its electric-red sign that said AMBULANCES. With the sirens off, as we waited for the world's slowest garage door to peel open, it was eerily quiet. We looked at each other, anxiety high. The patient was only forty years old and had collapsed in front of his wife, who immediately began CPR while his daughter dialled 911. If anyone could be saved, it was this man. I zapped him again as the back doors of the truck swung open.

After an hour or so, the electrocardiogram was flat. The emergency doctor placed an ultrasound probe on the patient's chest, angling it upwards to show an image of a heart that was still. The only thing left on the list of possible causes was a massive blockage high up in one of the two main coronary arteries that deliver oxygenated blood to the ventricles of the heart. Back in 2007, there was no fix for that. And the dozen or so professionals in the resuscitation bay looked around at each other, drenched in sweat, and sighed or frowned or closed their eyes or did whatever they did when a person was dead-dead. Then I went and got a latte, because I was exhausted and there were still nine hours left in my shift.

AS A PARAMEDIC, I always felt limited: limited by my training, by my equipment, by the ridiculous rules that seemed to be written to make my shifts in the field feel like a job in a cubicle. I hated the feeling of dropping off a critically sick patient in an ER, never to hear of them again. Was my diagnosis right? Did my treatment work? As a paramedic, I never really knew.

I was hungry for more than I could offer in my role. I didn't dislike being a paramedic; in fact, I loved it, and I often think it was the best job I've ever had. Whether on an ambulance roaming the streets of Toronto or in a helicopter two thousand feet over rural Ontario, I had found my calling. But something was missing, and I wanted to find it.

My mentors sensed this, and one of them, Al Craig, a paramedic who rose through the ranks to become deputy chief of the paramedic service in Toronto, issued a warning to me: if I didn't apply to medical school, I'd never forgive myself. Al had never done it, despite having a masters degree and quickly rising through the ranks in municipal management. When he spoke of what his life could have been, his regret was palpable, a regret he hoped I would never feel myself. It always seemed a bit unwarranted for Al to raise doctors on a pedestal when it could be argued that his own career, building one of Canada's best ambulance services, had saved more lives than most doctors could in a lifetime. But I knew paramedics were often disparaged by emergency department doctors and nurses, and Al had a lot more years than I had of being subjected to that.

Al, bald and aging, had a face that folded in such a way as to accentuate his eyes, giving him a puppy-dog gaze. You could say no to him, but not forever. He played the long game, building his argument over time at dinners and on flights to conferences and on phone calls that were supposed to be about clinical and research projects. He eventually framed my application to medical school as a favour to his younger self.

After years of prodding, I eventually gave in and submitted an application to med school. Every hopeful candidate was required to complete an online personality assessment that involved watching a series of videos that posed ethical and moral dilemmas and saying how you would respond to them. In the fall of 2010, when I was supposed to log in to complete the assessment, I was backpacking through Morocco, and despite my efforts to book a decent Wi-Fi-equipped hotel in Tangier, a glitch meant the videos wouldn't play, and I was left to describe how I would respond to scenarios I never actually saw. At the time, I was more pissed off that I'd spent forty euros on a hotel instead of four euros on a hostel bed than I was at losing out at my chance (and Al's) to go to medical school.

But Al convinced me to give it another go. I applied again the following year, and this time I was travelling through western China when my online assessment was scheduled. As a young paramedic, October was the only month I could ever get four weeks' vacation because, like everything in paramedicine, the only thing people judge you on is your seniority as published by the union, and my relatively low seniority severely limited my freedom to schedule vacation time. It's not like you can walk into a Starbucks and get free Wi-Fi connectivity in the People's Republic, so once again, I would have to chance a hotel. This time, I was able to scope out the Sheraton in Chengdu.

Fortunately, the connection held up, and I was able to watch the videos and declare that, no, I would not be pressing charges against the impoverished mother who stole a jar of baby food for her infant, and no, I would not be accepting the trip to Hawaii to endorse a new drug, and yes, I would be a good team player on a mission to Mars, because I was hilarious and agreeable and a problem-solver and other buzzwords that couldn't possibly predict if I'd actually be a good doctor but that could get me through to an interview to medical school.

I was accepted to McMaster University medical school in May 2012 and three months later moved to Hamilton, an hour west of Toronto and affectionately known as the armpit of Ontario because its dwindling steel mills once left a hazy stench over the city. People who are born in Hamilton say it's the Brooklyn of Toronto, but that seems delusional to anyone who has actually been to Brooklyn. At best, Truth and Synonym, my hipster coffee shops, could be transplanted to Brooklyn, but that's about the only similarity between the two.

I dropped down to part-time paramedic work, and some months later I quit the ground ambulance job to be able to meet the minimum shift requirements of my helicopter bosses, a job I favoured between the two because working on a helicopter that lands in the middle of a highway is about the coolest thing anyone can do. I was able to cling to that gig until April 2018, when the demands of residency were just too much and I was "asked" to quit.

As I progressed through my training, my title kept advancing: a student becomes a clerk, who becomes an intern, who becomes a junior resident, who becomes a senior resident, who becomes a fellow. Eventually, I reached the coveted title of Attending, which means you are a fully fledged consultant, an expert in your discipline and someone who, ostensibly, is no longer required to work eighty hours each week.

As I rose through the ranks, so too did my level of responsibility. With this rise comes an inherent discomfort, a distrust of yourself to get it right every time. This imposter syndrome is well documented, but there's no effective cure. As the situations I had to solve got more complex, the feeling I was an imposter strengthened, and I longed for those days as a paramedic when I could call a doctor for reassurance—and to diffuse my own responsibility for a situation. But now there was no one to call. The decision to declare death was now mine alone, and I never came across a patient who met the criteria of Policy 4.4. My paramedic friends never brought a single one of those to the emergency room—those patients were left in the field for the coroner's office to collect, dead-dead. My days of seeing death as black and white were over; it was shades of grey, and there was no policy manual to guide me.

In the ER, I found I could go further to reverse death than I ever could before. Most of the time in the ER, you go through the motions — the way you do as a paramedic — your gut instincts validating the algorithms taped on the walls of every resus bay I've ever seen: cycles of CPR, attempts at defibrillation, adrenalin every five minutes or so. It's remarkably routine. Ten minutes in, you tend to know. A flat line, a weak squiggle, a pathetic tracing of a heart that is too sick to beat. As the minutes tick by, the energy in the room starts to fade. Then you pause, look into the creepily open eyes of your patient, and purse your lips. At least, that's what one of the nurses told me I do. She said everyone has a tell, like a card player who's bluffing. I squeeze my lips together, more so on the left side, and it pushes the tip of my nose slightly to the right. That's how she'd know I was out of ideas, out of hope.

Half the time, I don't bother to announce time of death the way they do on television — my team knows the fight's over, and whoever is charting is just as capable of looking at their watch as I am. We all step out of the room and resume our other duties.

But there are always those cases that remind you why you're awake at 3 a.m. surrounded by cranky walk-ins with the flu and chronic back pain and vomiting induced by marijuana. Those cases where the algorithm, the routine, is tossed aside and you keep going and going and going. Where the energy doesn't dim, and no one thinks of quitting. Those cases, which might be one in ten patients, are why people work in demoralizing emergency rooms around the world. Those saves—we call them ROSCS (return of spontaneous circulation)—are joyful moments.

AFTER A FEW YEARS of residency in the ER, I felt the same grumbling discontent I'd felt as a paramedic; I wanted to know more, do more, and see people through the next stage of their illness. I mentioned this to one of my mentors, Randy Wax. Randy is an endlessly optimistic, portly man with a high-pitched voice who seems to channel the Energizer bunny. Those traits make him an incredible leader and teacher, which is why he used to be an esteemed professor in medical education at the University of Toronto before accepting dual directorships in education and critical care at a large community hospital to the east of the city.

I first met Randy in 2007, when he showed up to train the class of future flight paramedics I had joined. As if all of his current roles weren't enough, Randy wished he could be a paramedic, and as a consolation prize he manned the phones at the helicopter dispatch centre where paramedics called in for guidance using crackly satellite phones.

Randy told me that spending time in the ICU would quench my thirst. There, I could see the full spectrum of critical illness, from the moment patients arrived off the ER elevator to the moment they either died or got better. The dichotomy of outcomes in the ICU is striking, even more so than in the emergency department. As Randy puts it, you either "resuscitate or palliate" — opposite ends of the spectrum, both of which are somehow, he assured me, equally rewarding.

I began moonlighting in Randy's ICU, working twenty-four hour shifts on weekends and loving every minute of it. I'd race between beds, managing strokes, heart attacks, and the most adrenalin-pumping situation of them all: code blues.

I DON'T REALLY NEED to explain what a code blue is. Popularized by television, it's the highest priority of announcement over the hospital PA system. I used to be rattled when the words blared out of the overhead speakers because code blues aren't as smooth and straightforward as they seem on TV. They are generally described as shit-shows. And the more code blues I saw, the more distressed I became. There was so much variation in how these codes went that I became compelled to study them.

When I was doing my master's degree in science at one of Toronto's trauma centres, I was responsible for studying the behaviours of code blue teams made up of doctors, nurses, respiratory therapists, and pharmacists. I would sift through computer data, trying to understand why there were delays in giving drugs or shocks, any hint of process problems that could be improved to save lives. I carried a code blue pager that was so large it resembled an old Sony Walkman, and within a year I had responded to over one hundred code blues. As a paramedic, my job had been to lead code blues, my eyes on the patient and their heart rhythm; as a researcher, my job was to stand in the corner and stay quiet, assessing how the team performed, all but ignoring the patient.

I quickly became frustrated by the codes. Second-year internal medicine residents were in charge of blues, and their performance was somewhat sub-par; you can't really blame them as for many it was one of the first, and last, codes they would ever run. I got into the habit of leaving the codes as quickly as possible, often before they were resolved; my heart just couldn't take it. Paramedics practice in simulators for years to earn the privilege of running resuscitations, but at this hospital, as it is in every other university hospital I've worked at, it seemed that taking a weekend course was all you needed to be put in charge of what is more often than not the end of someone's life; the intense simulator time just wasn't required.

My experiences drove me to dedicate my science efforts to improving how people perform resuscitations, with the idealistic dream that everyone whose heart stopped could get the most thorough, evidence-based, perfectly choreographed medical response possible — the best chance at a second life.

But as time went on, I began to realize something with startling clarity: there are people who shouldn't receive any resuscitation at all.

RANDY THOUGHT I HAD a knack for working in the ICU, and he began pushing me towards doing extra training to become dual qualified for both the emergency room and ICU, or "downstairs and upstairs" as he called it, reflecting the physical reality of most hospitals.

Having trained in Pittsburgh, or "Pitt" as it's famously known in the medical world, Randy encouraged me to head south of the 49th parallel for my fellowship. After interviewing at Stanford University Medical Center, it was clear to me that it would be my next home: the ICU director who interviewed me has a Ph.D. in palliative care, and our "interview" was more of a jam on the death dilemma.

So I packed up, deferred my job as an attending physician in an emergency room in Toronto, and booked one of the last direct flights to San Francisco—the route was being cancelled because of the coronavirus pandemic. Fernando, my boyfriend (now my fiancé), dropped me off at the airport, and after a long embrace I headed inside the terminal to continue my pursuit of learning how to save people's lives—and address my sense of discomfort around what to do when saving a life is unrealistic.

As I continued to train, saving lives seemed only half the equation I needed to solve to be an effective critical care doctor. I also needed to find an approach to the patient who, no matter what I did, was going to die. My angst was rooted in two fears: one, that I wasn't good enough to save their life, that I was somehow missing something that could be fixed; and two, that even when there was nothing left to fix, I couldn't somehow navigate a path to their dignified death.

It might seem odd that this would be on my list of learning objectives eight years after starting medical school and fifteen years after I began work as a paramedic. Seeing how over fifty million people die every year around the world, you'd think we'd know everything there is to know about death. Yet we don't really know much at all; with each advance in technology and medical science, perhaps we know less than ever before. As Elisabeth Kübler-Ross, the Swiss-American pioneer in this area of study, said after spending years interviewing the dying in hospitals, death is the "greatest mystery in science," a statement as true today as it was when she said it over fifty years ago.

Now, I encounter almost daily situations where the life I'm entrusted with can't be saved, but where death is anything but black and white. Medical technology that replaces certain organs has created a confusing reality: a patient may be dead but have a beating heart, while another may be playing chess but have no heartbeat at all.

I CAN'T RECALL A time as a paramedic where I pronounced someone dead without complete confidence. If I couldn't get your heart started in your living room or bedroom or bathroom (where many people seem to die, a surprising number somehow wedged between the toilet and the wall), no one else was going to be able to.

You were dead, and I'd be confident calling it. Families would accept it. But the difference in the field was that there wasn't any life-sustaining technology to remove; I would make the decision, independent of the family, and turn off the flatlining heart monitor.

It was easy. But my experiences as a physician slowly eroded, rather than reinforced, my confidence in diagnosing death.

I REMEMBER ONE SHIFT in the pediatric ICU that was particularly jarring. A young boy, eleven years old, had a severe kidney infection at a community hospital about an hour's drive away. He arrived by helicopter in dire shape. The infection had started in his abdomen, triggering the body's immune system. The immune system went haywire, generating chemicals meant to help but that were actually doing more harm than good. His blood pressure became dangerously low, so low his brain wasn't getting enough oxygen to feed its delicate neurons. His lungs began to dysfunction, requiring us to use a ventilator to push oxygen into his bloodstream across the gossamer-thin-walled alveoli that swell like bunches of grapes at the end of the air passageways.

His body wouldn't respond to any of our therapies. The laboratory data kept getting worse, and you could see colour and life drain from his body.

Around midnight, my boss said, "He's probably dead." She was referring to his brain being dead, which is how many ICU patients die, though we keep them attached to machines and medicine drips that can keep hearts beating and lungs breathing long after the brain has shut down.

"We'll test his brain stem in the morning. I'm going home to get some sleep," she said plainly, before walking out through the wide, automatic doors of the icu, leaving me to care for him, and eleven other children, until sunrise.

I was left to tend to a boy who we thought was dead, and if not, surely would be soon. The next morning, after we reviewed morning blood work and chest X-rays for the twelve patients in the unit, we tested his brain stem. A series of stimuli—rapid head motion, ice-cold water in the ear canal, trying to make him gag by shoving a suction catheter down his throat—had no effect and left us convinced.

The last step in declaring brain death is to turn off the ventilator and see if the brain triggers a breath. We waited for ten minutes, watching his carbon dioxide levels rise beyond the level that triggers a deep inspiration. His chest didn't move. He was dead. The time was 10:15 a.m.

I sat at a desk, filling out his death certificate, while the organ donation coordinator sat beside me making calls on her cellphone, trying to allocate his organs. The next morning, before the sun came up, I walked down to the operating room and helped cut out his heart. And then, twenty-eight hours or so after we figured he was probably dead, and sixteen hours after he was declared dead, he was dead-dead. Except for his heart, which is beating in a chest somewhere in Alberta. His heart is very much alive.

THAT ENTIRE EXPERIENCE WAS very strange to me, back in 2014. It was the first time I had been present when someone was declared brain dead. For all the times I had pronounced people dead in my paramedic days, I had never had to be so meticulous, so detailed, in making sure death had been realized.

But as my training progressed, brain death cases became a relief. With the diagnosis of brain death came an end to our resuscitation efforts, as the paradigm shifted from saving a patient's life to saving the lives of those depending on viable organs. It was definitive, final; it was over.

The real struggle for doctors like me lies in those who aren't brain dead but who are terribly sick, the ones who require machine after machine to stay alive but will not recover, at least not in a meaningful way.

During the coronavirus pandemic, I cared for hundreds of people sickened by the virus to the extent that they required life support. A little more than half survived to leave my ICU; the rest died slowly, over weeks, as the virus shredded their lungs. The body's response to the coronavirus was often unhelpful. Chemicals released by the immune system would cause the sponge-like lungs to stiffen into crunchy steel wool. Once that occurred, lung transplantation was the only path to recovery, and most patients aren't candidates.

Worse, there were way more potential candidates than donor lungs.

To guide us, experts devised criteria for lung transplant candidates. It was pretty easy to end up excluded. Being overweight often disqualified patients because overweight COVID-19 patients often had much worse outcomes; virus-shredded lungs have trouble expanding against a massive belly, and it was hard to heal.

This put us in a tough spot: after three or four weeks, we could tell which patients were on the path to recovery and which were not going to make it. Backup plans had been written at the highest levels of government that would allow us to unilaterally remove these patients from ventilators if we didn't have enough machines to go around. Fortunately, this worst-case scenario never happened where I work.

But in many ways, a policy might have been helpful; for many patients whose chances of survival were next to zero, families and medical teams alike struggled to accept the inevitable outcome.

I remember one thirty-year-old who, in the peak of the pandemic, was too far gone to save, ineligible for additional machines and transplants. There was no way out. Day after day, he would have life-threatening episodes where the breathing machine couldn't deliver enough oxygen to him; we would rush to apply safety gear, run into the room, and begin manually inflating his lungs with an Ambu bag—essentially a bellows for your lungs. Sometimes for over an hour, until our hands would cramp, we would have to bag his lungs before he settled back on to the machine. The whole time I was wondering what on earth we were doing.

We would use words on the phone with his family that were direct but not quite crystal clear: "He's doing worse today" or "I'm very worried he won't make it," but never "This is the end" or "He's about to die." So for days longer than we should have, we kept putting him through the pains and trials of modern intensive care.

Eventually, his heart stopped. Despite the fact that chest compressions would not help, we did them anyway, because a note from a medical student said his family wanted "everything done."

I'm glad I wasn't at work when he coded. I'm not sure I could have stood there and watched my colleagues pound on his chest. I know a few doctors who just wouldn't bother; they'd just stop, and it would be over. But the culture at many hospitals is that more is more, and most people in the ICU get extreme measures even when everyone knows they won't work.

This scene has been replayed so many times during the COVID-19 pandemic. Too many doctors just won't say "There is no way out." Many of these patients are full code, meaning the medical team is compelled to maximally resuscitate them with techniques that just aren't meant for people with end-stage lung disease. CPR and rescue breaths work when someone has been pulled unresponsive from a swimming pool or their heart stops at the casino, but not when other organs are shutting down. When the heart stops because the lungs are broken, coding someone does nothing but ensure an undignified, miserable end. Based on common practice in Canada, where I trained in the ER, I eventually stopped offering CPR to dying COVID-19 patients. That made many of my American peers—nurses, respiratory therapists, other doctors— profoundly unsettled. Some of us, myself included, wouldn't offer the full suite of resuscitation procedures—as one ICU director said, "We don't offer futile care." But others, stuck in the do-everything mentality, run the code, sometimes for thirty or forty minutes, throwing the kitchen sink at someone in their final moments.

The implications of this go beyond wasted syringes and defibrillator pads. Families would be ushered away, chaos would fill what should be a peaceful, reverent place, and staff would have visceral reactions, using words like "cruel" and "unethical" to describe the final efforts expended on a patient. It was a lose-lose-lose scenario.

But it doesn't have to be that way.

IN THE ICU, death is not always as certain as it was for the thirty-year-old with horrible COVID-19 and shredded lungs. Sometimes there's a chance, and when there is, doctors tend to paint a simplified picture. We say the odds may not be great, but there is a chance. "A chance at what?" is something we aren't good at describing.

For some, it may be a chance at full recovery. For others, it's a chance to be in a nursing facility attached to feeding tubes and breathing machines. But when people decide to roll the dice and ask that "everything" medically possible be done, they do so without knowing what that might mean.

When there is a choice to be made, it is not mine alone, but I play an integral role: my honest and clear assessment, and how I communicate it to loved ones, can ease the decision to let go of someone in a controlled, peaceful way. If I do this right, and families process the details with an open mind, an assured death can be beautiful, tender, and comfortable. It can bring peace and closure. It can avoid the chaos, the broken ribs, and the existential distress that comes with coding someone who is too far gone to benefit from modern medicine.

But too often there is ambiguity, and it usually leads to decisions being deferred, the direct consequence of which is more suffering. If I cry at work, it's usually after conversations where I have to look families in the eyes but can't quite bring myself to tell them what they ought to hear. Technology can prevent death from coming too soon, but it can also delay its timely arrival. With the power granted by advanced technology to cheat death, doctors must also have the wisdom to know when and how to wield it, because death will come for all of us. How to achieve a timely death isn't really taught in medical schools or spoken about in hospital hallways, and it has become a critical gap in our culture. That gap led me to write this book so I could come to some sort of peace myself about how my efforts to save lives might somehow be backfiring.

I'm working in the grey zone between life and death, and it's an agonizing place to be.

CHAPTER 2

A Brief History of Death

IF WE GO BACK a century, doctors weren't typically presented with a dilemma when patients neared death. It just kind of happened. Lungs would stop breathing, hearts would stop pumping, and there was nothing anyone could do about it. It was so common, it almost always happened in the same bed a person had slept in their whole life, surrounded by their family.

Sometimes I long for those simpler days. No laboratory tests or diagnostic imaging or surgical implants. Physicians were armed with a few concoctions and devices, but they relied mostly on their wit.

I figured that if I was having trouble finding my way through the death dilemma, I should start with a look back at simpler times, before machines could play understudy to leading organs. But it turns out that those simpler times were more complicated than one might think. Before the mid-nineteenth century, back when physicians rarely had medical degrees and often had no training at all, history is riddled with stories — some accurate, some folklore — of people declared dead who then woke up, sometimes at their own funerals.

Such errors were frequent enough, it seems, that people went to extreme lengths to prevent being buried alive. Various rituals became established to prevent the frightening possibility. In ancient times, the Greeks would cut off a finger to check for a reaction, while Hebrews would wait for bodies to decay.

Fear of misdiagnosing death persisted as a social phenomenon right into the 1800s, leading the Victorians to a common preoccupation: the danger of a premature burial. This anxiety, which peaked during cholera epidemics, is articulated in Edgar Allan Poe's 1844 horror story "The Premature Burial," in which the narrator's fear of being buried alive becomes a phobia. His dread centres on what doctors at the time termed "catalepsy," a condition where people appeared dead but were in fact comatose. So haunted were the Victorians by this possibility that they founded the Society for the Prevention of People Being Buried Alive.

Strange workarounds ensued, such as burying the dead with shovels so they could dig themselves out of their own graves, placing glass over the deceased's face so nightwatchmen could monitor for signs of life, and installing pipes from buried coffins to the surface and employing observers to listen for wails from the revived.

By the late 1800s, many were opting not to be buried at all until their bodies displayed assurances of death, primarily putrefaction. When he died in 1852, Arthur Wellesley, 1st Duke of Wellington, laid in state for two months after his death, reportedly out of an abundance of caution to ensure he was in fact dead.

IT OCCURRED TO ME that, with guidance, these historic tales of death, near death, and dying might help lead me towards some answers to the modern death dilemma. But searching for a death historian is not as easy at it sounds. I guess it's not really something you put on a business card or hire a search engine optimization company to emphasize. Eventually, however, I came across Stephen Berry, a professor in the history department at the University of Georgia. I saw he had published a book titled *The Historian as Death Investigator* in 2011. I had found my man.

Steve had just finished a new book, on death registries, called *Counting the Dead*, and was happy to help me with the death dilemma. After describing my conundrum and asking him to help set me on a path to enlightenment, he said, with the excitement of a university professor at the front of a lecture auditorium, "We only have to go back two hundred years!" (What a relief!)

Two hundred years ago, Steve explained, when nearly everyone died in their living room or their bed, they fulfilled "the most important role of their lives: they showed other people how to die." As Steve explains it, when death was a common thing to witness, it was thus somewhat normalized. It wouldn't be unusual for a mother to bear six or eight children but have only two or three survive to adult age. Infections, accidents, and violence killed many adults in their twenties and thirties. A simple skin puncture could get infected, and in the absence of antibiotics, people would die of sepsis.

Doctors had a paucity of pharmaceuticals and medical interventions at their disposal. Things that today I can't imagine someone dying of, like postpartum bleeding or a dental abscess, could be deadly. This meant that, throughout your life, siblings, uncles, aunts, friends, and others around you would die, and when they did, there was a good chance you'd be there when it happened. There was a fear of death, but no denial that it would come.

Death pervaded so much of life, Steve told me, that the Shaker sect was in part born out of it. Ann Lee, the daughter of a blacksmith in Manchester, England, and one of the community's earliest members, had lost all four of her children to early death from various causes. It's believed that this cumulative loss led the founders of the Shakers to believe that you shouldn't have children at all. The group's members practised celibacy and were against procreation.

Infant and child mortality really dragged down life expectancy. Global life expectancy in the nineteenth century was around thirty years, but by 2000 it was nearly seventy; today, the residents of some countries, like Switzerland and Japan, enjoy life expectancies of over eighty years. Steve credits advances in public health and medicine to the doubling of life expectancy in this time. "It happened relatively overnight," he told me.

Steve was sympathetic to the death dilemma I was experiencing. He reassured me that technology had complicated things. While advances in science and medicine brought longer life expectancy and were welcomed, they brought with them a challenge too: the medicalization of the dying process. Before the mid-twentieth century, pronouncement of death wasn't so much a formal process as it was a natural conclusion. "Pa would just die in his bed," according to Steve. The grey zone I was caught up in simply didn't exist for most of human history, he made clear; death could not be deferred. It came when it came, and that was that.

I DECIDED TO DIG into the reasons life expectancy doubled between 1850 and 1950, a light-speed improvement over the millennia before. The idea that people were living longer meant that the average person saw fewer deaths throughout their life among family and friends, and that societal shift would, I figured, be relevant to the death dilemma.

Vaccines, antibiotics, and public health measures like clean water and simple hygiene saw to it that, in the space of decades, common killers vanished. A Hungarian obstetrician, Ignaz Semmelweis, found in 1847 that when he washed his hands with antiseptic between delivering babies, he could virtually eliminate "childbed fever," which, unknown to anyone at the time, was caused by the bacteria streptococcus.

At the Vienna General Hospital, where Semmelweis was employed, one in ten women would die of the fever shortly after giving birth. Handwashing was infrequent, and obstetricians would often deliver babies after conducting autopsies of other new mothers who had died of the infection. After the introduction of chlorine hand wash, mortality of postpartum women fell tenfold, to one percent. Similar results occurred when Semmelweis moved to hospitals in Budapest and Zurich, but it would be a few decades later, when Louis Pasteur published his germ theory, that the reason chlorine reduced deaths would begin to be understood.

Seven years after Semmelweis first started using chlorine, another pioneering doctor, John Snow, was tracing deaths attributed to cholera in London. By mapping the deaths, Snow traced them to their point of highest density in the Soho district. On a hunch, he removed the pump handle from a communal water source, and cholera deaths dropped. This eventually led to the discovery that the drinking water responsible for much of the outbreak was being pumped from the Thames downstream of a sewage facility contaminated by cholera-laden feces, a reality that contributed to Pasteur's later elucidation that "germs" were responsible for much human suffering.

So influential were Snow and Semmelweis to advancing human health that there are monuments erected in their honour, and being a nerdy doctor, I've tracked them both down. Semmelweis has been declared the "saviour of mothers," and the very handle John Snow removed from the pump in Soho is enclosed in a glass case at the London School of Hygiene and Tropical Medicine, where I trained in infectious disease and public health. My classmates and I clamoured around the handle when we first saw it. No inscription was needed to explain its significance; we just knew it was the famous Broad Street pump handle.

The advent of vaccines and antibiotics round out innovations that, when combined with advances in public health and hygiene like the ones I've described above, saw death rates drop precipitously. While this is cause for celebration, it created a new problem for doctors and society. People were living longer.

BY THE 1950s, advances in industry and the post–Second World War surge in technological innovation were leading to an explosion of medical technologies and pharmaceuticals.

The previous hundred years had seen to it that mothers stopped contracting streptococcus during labour, or that those who did were saved by penicillin; cholera outbreaks were squashed by epidemiologists armed with maps; smallpox was on its way to being eradicated; and in 1952, the polio vaccine was invented. But there was still little doctors could do to stop an imminent death. While society and medicine advanced, the declaration of death remained relatively low-tech: a physician would look for respirations and feel for a pulse. If neither was found, the physician would declare death, much as had been the case for centuries.

Steve Berry agreed with my assessment that the critical advances in resuscitation technology of the '50s and '60s were a moment of confluence: people were living longer, we were becoming less comfortable with death, and we were more capable of prolonging life artificially. It was the perfect recipe for creating a world where people, and their doctors, would forget how to die.

CHAPTER 3

A Modern Day Disruption

WE'VE ESTABLISHED THAT, for millennia, people died without much fuss. Little could be done to alter the course of nature until the nineteenth century, when human life expectancy suddenly doubled. But if that hundred years saw rapid progression, the last half-century or so, from the 1950s to the present, has seen a lightning-fast technological revolution in medicine and science. Modern medicine can now subdue, if not cure, so many diseases that were once death sentences. And in doing so, it has, in every way, disrupted death and dying.

Medical students now learn radiological anatomy. I remember sliding a piezoelectric crystal probe around a fellow student's abdomen and staring at shades of grey on an ultrasound screen as I tried to interpret a liver or a kidney from the snowstorm of pixels in front of me. I spent hours in dark rooms staring at CT scans of brains, trying to learn the difference between grey matter, which looks white, and white matter, which looks grey. I was tested on ventilator modes, cardioversion energy settings, and dialysis fluids. And, of course, each time I rotated through a new hospital, I would have to learn how to pull up X-rays, enter prescriptions, and review laboratory results on a suite of glitchy software platforms.

Technology in health care is ubiquitous. Most of it has simply replaced something that once existed on paper or film as we shifted to a digital world, but it is the advance of *mechanical* technology that has thrown us into the death dilemma. The innovation of the 1950s would create an arms race of sorts for engineers and doctors to build ever-more-sophisticated devices to support the dying. I wanted to understand how it came to be that I could replace the delicate work of human organs with machines. It was time to find the innovators, the inventors, the engineers who made these marvellous devices that are causing me so much angst.

I DECIDED TO START with the most consequential device of them all, the one that can keep oxygen flowing into the body to sustain cells that, if deprived of the simple molecule for just a few minutes, will die.

I called Arthur Slutsky, an engineer, innovator, and pulmonologist who is famous for holding a number of patents for ventilators. Art was my boss's boss's boss when I was completing my master's degree in resuscitation science at the University of Toronto in 2006, back when I was running around a hospital observing code blues. Art graciously took my call, even though it had been over a decade since we last spoke.

"It started before the 1950s," he told me, and he described the impacts of the polio epidemic in the 1930s and '40s. That epidemic, he explained, brought about a major shift in how doctors viewed breathing. Before the 1930s, physicians hadn't really understood much about why people breathe. They assumed the rhythmic movement of the chest somehow supported blood circulation. Negative-pressure devices like the iron lung device could support a polio patient's rhythmic chest movements to a point.

With the spread of polio, that began to change. Doctors could now perform various chemical tests on patients, such as bicarbonate levels in blood serum. At the time, bicarbonate was associated with the kidneys, which excrete it in urine or resorb it into the bloodstream. But with polio, which weakened and paralyzed muscles responsible for breathing, like the diaphragm, bicarbonate levels would rise. Assuming at first that the kidneys were being killed off by the polio virus, doctors took years to realize that respiratory failure was in fact the culprit.

As the lungs fail, the acid carbon dioxide accumulates in the body because it can't escape through exhaling lungs. The kidneys, in response to the acidification of the blood, retain bicarbonate, a base, in an effort to equal out the body's pH.

Once doctors realized that rises in bicarbonate were caused by failing lungs rather than failing kidneys, they doubled down on ventilation devices, expanding from negative-pressure devices like the iron lung to positive-pressure ventilators that would generate more gas exchange; by blowing air in, carbon dioxide will be blown out.

Art told me about what he called an inflection point. In 1952, when a large outbreak of paralytic polio occurred in Copenhagen, a physician there decided to start ventilating patients. At first, he recruited medical students to manually blow air into the patients' lungs using rubber bags, like the Ambu bag I used when I worked on ambulances. In a landmark publication, he was able to show that in July of that year, 80 percent of paralytic polio patients would die of the infectious disease. But in August, when he arranged to have patients ventilated, only 40 percent died.

When the *Lancet* published data showing ventilation could cut polio deaths in half, the technique was quickly mimicked around the world. "It was very dramatic, literally overnight," Art said of the impact of the Copenhagen study. But there were two problems: patients needed to be ventilated for weeks, and medical students needed to sleep. (To this day, many physicians believe medical students don't need to sleep.)

"Hand-bagging" a patient is hard work; every medical student is still made to practise the skill in the operating room, using one hand to seal a plastic mask around the patient's mouth and nose (far more difficult than you might think) while extending the wrist to lift the jaw, and thus the tongue, off the back of the throat so air can flow freely. The other hand then squeezes a large rubber sac of air every five seconds or so. It's tricky for first-time baggers; every medical student is forced to prove their technique under the peering glare of an anesthesiologist.

But it's not just tricky for the uninitiated; the task is so challenging, in fact, that I've gotten into some serious hot water when "bagging" a patient was difficult. Beards pose a problem, as you can't get a good seal with the mask, and people with large heads and necks sometimes require two hands — or even two people — to lift the jaw and unobstruct the tongue from the back of the mouth. In one case, shortly after becoming an attending, I briefly lost a patient's pulse because I couldn't bag her. (My own pulse at the time was through the roof.)

The skill, needless to say, is one we don't take for granted. After just a few minutes of bagging someone, your hands start to cramp, your wrist gets weak, and the novice student is sure to get a stern correction from the attending anesthesiologist. Eventually, once satisfied that the pupil appreciates the pitfalls of the technique, the boss relents and attaches the patient to a ventilator, relieving the medical student's aching hand from duty.

Enter Forrest Bird, a Second World War pilot from Massachusetts with a knack for innovation. Bird's early foray into ventilators began after examining a German Junkers Ju 88 warplane. At the time, American pilots were limited in how high they could fly, because even though they used oxygen masks, they would lose consciousness over twenty-eight thousand feet. The Ju 88 had a mask that delivered pressurized oxygen, allowing pilots to fly higher—up to thirty-five thousand feet, about the elevation a Boeing 777 from New York to Paris would fly.

Fascinated by respiratory physiology, Bird applied to medical school after the war. When a friend's father began to decompensate from emphysema, he used a doorknob from a hardware store to create a device that could provide adjustable airflow. From there, he used strawberry shortcake tins and a regulator from a pilot G-suit to create a model positive-pressure ventilator.

Bird wasn't the only person innovating ventilators in the 1950s; similar efforts were underway in Scandinavia, the United Kingdom, and the United States. But Bird's invention was remarkable, because it was cheap and easy to make. By 1957, he had created six prototypes before the Bird Mark 7 ventilator hit the market. Similar devices proliferated in a matter of just a few years, and by the 1960s, ventilators were standard in hospitals around the world.

Ventilators were a game-changer. The act of breathing could now be fully automated, and patients who required the devices were eventually sequestered together, forming the first intensive care units.

In the same year the Bird Mark 7 ventilator was commercialized, an accidental discovery in Baltimore, Maryland, changed the game again.

IN 2010, I RODE an elevator with Guy Knickerbocker, who was seventy-eight years old at the time. I stood there, silent, screaming on the inside, as if I'd just seen Brad Pitt circa *Fight Club* standing in line next to me at Starbucks. That's because I was, at the time, an up-and-coming CPR (cardiopulmonary resuscitation) scientist, and I was standing a few feet away from the guy who, fifty years earlier, had discovered CPR. Prior to Knickerbocker, you could pump all the oxygen into the lungs you wanted, but if the heart wasn't beating, there was no circulating blood to take it to the organs (unless doctors cracked your chest open and manually massaged your heart, which, you can imagine, is a bit of a to-do).

We both stepped out of the elevator onto the ninth floor of a Dallas hotel. He turned left, and I turned right. When I got to my room, my trance broke and I cursed at the missed opportunity. We were both in the hotel for a conference celebrating the fiftieth anniversary of CPR's first use to restart a stopped heart, and Dr. Knickerbocker, who was an electrical engineer, was receiving a lifetime achievement award for his contributions to medicine.

Later that evening, on my way to dinner, luck was on my side: Knickerbocker was waiting patiently when I arrived at the elevators. Having frozen up once, I wasn't going to give up the moment. I introduced myself and asked if I might steal a few moments of his time. He happily accepted my invitation, and we sat on a couch in the elevator lobby and chatted. At first it was surreal; my journalism instincts deserted me entirely, and

I failed to take notes or record our chat. I have had to fact-check my memory with accounts in medical journals to reconstruct what was, I guarantee you, the most inspiring conversation I've ever had.

Knickerbocker was a graduate student at Johns Hopkins University, working in a cardiology lab funded by the Edison Electric Institute to create a portable defibrillator to apply to utility workers who were being electrocuted on the job. Back then, defibrillators weighed over two hundred pounds and had to be wheeled around on frames the size of modern dishwashers.

To do this, Knickerbocker and his lab assistant induced ventricular fibrillation in dogs, then shocked them back into a normal heart rhythm. When you're in V-fib, you don't have a pulse (neither do dogs). Knickerbocker found he had about five minutes to shock a dog before the heart would die from a lack of oxygen and enter asystole, or flatline, at which point the animal was a goner.

One evening, after inducing V-fib in a dog, Knickerbocker turned to reach for the defibrillator paddles. Except the defibrillator wasn't there.

Knickerbocker began to fret. The defibrillator had been borrowed by a lab on the fifth floor, seven floors beneath them. In the 1950s, elevators weren't exactly fast, and Knickerbocker knew it would take more than five minutes to fetch the giant device.

That's when he remembered an observation in earlier defibrillations. The dogs had pressure monitors placed in their groin arteries, and Knickerbocker recalled that when the heavy metal paddles of the defibrillator were applied to the dogs' chests, before any shock was delivered, the pressure monitor would show a blip on the screen, like a spike on a seismograph during an earthquake. This indicated that the weight of the paddles caused a rush of blood to the groin, likely by ejecting blood out of the chest.

Knickerbocker thought fast. He instructed his assistant to press repeatedly on the dog's chest during the twenty minutes it took him to fetch the defibrillator. (He told me he ran down the stairs but had to wait for the elevator to bring him back up to the twelfth floor.) The dog survived. While defibrillation and rescue breathing had been experimented with in some form for centuries, this was the first time anyone had documented that external forces could cause the heart to beat. They went on to establish that they could leave a dog in V-fib for an hour and, as long as CPR was being done, defibrillation would still be successful. Knickerbocker shared his findings, and a year later CPR was being tested on humans. When Knickerbocker and his colleagues published their findings in the summer of 1960, CPR quickly became a medical standard for patients whose hearts had stopped. "We had found a way to slow down the dying process," he told the BBC in a 2015 interview, and I'm quite sure, though not sure enough to say so without a reference, that he said the same thing to me.

EVEN AS KNICKERBOCKER WAS defibrillating dogs and Bird was building ventilators, there was no immediate sense of urgency to define death in light of these new technologies; defibrillation was rarely successful, and life on a ventilator was short. People would either recover from their disease, as polio patients often did, or despite a ventilator, die in short order, as was the case in brain trauma and severe pneumonia. Besides, the sickest patients often didn't make it to a hospital where these devices could be applied.

But as defibrillators became smaller and CPR was taught to medical students around the world, and as ventilators became commonplace, doctors began to appreciate the lifesaving implications of applying invasive therapies to people on the brink of death. By the end of the 1960s, the word *resuscitation* was mainstream, and intensive care units had been established in most hospitals for diseases other than just polio. A lack of breathing or a stopped heart no longer signified death. Now, when faced with a dying patient, doctors could actually do something.

It became increasing clear that rapid actions, aided by new technologies, could save people's lives — or at least delay their deaths. Hospitals began to organize teams to resuscitate patients. Emergency doctors emerged as specialists, code blue teams became standard, and ICUs became beacons of hope. While engineers and doctors raced to develop more advanced technologies and techniques to resuscitate people admitted to hospital, another race was on to bring resuscitation out of the hospital and into the streets, where people were dying.

THE PROLIFERATION OF CARS had resulted in a spike in automobile-related fatalities, but most places lacked any organized ambulance system. If there was an ambulance service, you'd have to know the seven-digit phone number, assuming you could find a phone anywhere near the scene. This meant that people who suffered acute injury or sudden life-threatening illness faced dismal chances of surviving if they weren't already close a hospital. Recognizing this, governments began to formalize emergency care systems. In 1966, the U.S. National Academy of Sciences and the U.S. National Resource Council published the report *Accidental Death and Disability: The Neglected Disease of Modern Society*, setting off a flurry of activity to improve survival from traumatic injuries. As a result, the National Highway Traffic and Safety Administration was tasked with creating an ambulance network, and a pool of unemployed field medics who had returned from the Vietnam and Korean wars were some of the first to become "ambulance drivers."

Paramedics like me hate being called ambulance drivers. Driving is the mindless task we do when we aren't saving people's lives. But for the workers in the rapidly spreading ambulance services in the 1970s, it was very much a driving-focused job. The ambulances were essentially fancy taxis, vans with a stretcher in the back and lights on the roof. It was "scoop and run," the administering of "diesel therapy." But as ambulance workers got better training and became more sophisticated, emergency department care began to move to the streets. The modern defibrillator was now the size of a shoebox, not a dishwasher, and paramedic care extended beyond treating those with traumatic injuries to include heart and lung problems.

To find out more, I tracked down the first paramedic to use a defibrillator in Canada. It only took me about thirty minutes on Facebook. As it turns out, the person I was looking for was the father of Chris Bugelli, my partner on my first paramedic job, at Toronto's SkyDome stadium (now the Rogers Centre) in 2004, where we covered the crowd at Blue Jays baseball games.

John Bugelli started his career on the ambulances in Oshawa, where Randy Wax, the intensive care doctor who convinced me to do a fellowship in the U.S., now runs the ICU. Back in 1970, John's initial training was only six weeks long and consisted of "basic first aid and that type of crap," he told me, on an evening phone call from his home in Newcastle, Ontario. "We would do CPR, drive 'em to the hospital."

But then in 1975, Oshawa became the first ambulance service in the country to acquire defibrillators. The ambulance drivers in Oshawa were a young, enthusiastic group of guys based right at the Oshawa General Hospital, and in the ER were some equally young, enthusiastic emergency doctors. "We all got along," John said. "They said, 'If you wanna learn more, we'll teach you.' So we hung out, and they would show you something one or two times, then let you do it."

The doctors created a curriculum of sorts, and in the fall of 1975, they formally trained the first paramedics. Whether these were the first paramedics in the world to get this training is a matter of debate, and many places claim the honour—several countries were developing advanced resuscitation training for ambulance workers in the early 1970s. Before that, non-physician resuscitators were more or less limited to military combat.

Just a month after graduating in January 1976, John responded to a cardiac arrest in downtown Oshawa. "A guy had arrested in his car. We pulled him out, started doing the stuff, and I called it in." Back then, every action needed to be cleared by an emergency room doctor over the radio. "We defibrillated him once, and he came back."

"He came around fairly quick," John said. The man, a tailor, recovered after a few weeks in hospital. "It was basically shit luck," John told me with a wheezy laugh. Back then, the old-timers made fun of him and his eager workmates, regaling them with tales from the time before they even knew CPR, when the only decision to be made was whether to drive the bodies to an emergency room or a funeral home.

I brought up the death dilemma facing me in the tech-filled ICU and asked John what he thought about it. He told me what happened to him fourteen years ago. As it turns out, he is the beneficiary of defibrillation—seven shocks, to be exact.

After feeling chest pain, John knew he was having a heart attack. He called 911, and an ambulance rushed him to hospital, where his heart stopped. Once resuscitated, he was flown by helicopter to St. Michael's Hospital, in downtown Toronto. (It's possible, actually, that I was the one who flew him there, while training on the helicopters.)

I asked John what it was like to go from paramedic to patient.

"You know, I asked my doctor, 'Why did you shock me seven times? The protocol is for three or four.'" His doctor's response? "I could tell you were still fighting. As long you were fighting, I was going to fight too."

John told me a few jokes about his near-death experience, the type of jokes paramedics tell in the ambulance cab, ones that don't get repeated. Psychologists call this "dark humour," but most paramedics would argue that the levity keeps the darkness at bay.

As for the death dilemma, John's voice had a note of conviction when he answered: "The patient will tell you."

I thought he'd misunderstood my question and was about to say I was referring to ICU patients who are too sick to express their own wishes, but he wasn't finished.

"Even if they're unconscious, they can tell you themselves. I can't explain that. But when someone is ready to go, they are more relaxed. Have you noticed? It's like, 'Okay, I'm done.' In other words, they look like they don't have any fight left in them. As long as you can feel that fight is in the patient, you're going to keep going.

You'll be drenched in sweat, and you'll keep going."

I was excited. Finally, someone was able to explain a little of what I was trying to process in my role in a modern ICU, where the defibrillator is the simplest device we have. I asked John if he could teach a medical student what a person looks like when they are resigned to die.

"No," he said immediately. "You either have it or you don't."

TODAY, DIAGNOSING DEATH IS more complicated than ever, with life-sustaining technologies that go far beyond the simple bellows of prototypical ventilators and the crude zaps of joules delivered by defibrillators. Technology now exists that not only extends the shelf life of kidneys, hearts, intestines, and whatever the plural of *pancreas* is, but can replace organs' functions altogether.

For new doctors, these technologies are just a fact of life. Of course, most of my peers didn't spend ten years on the road as a paramedic, with only a defibrillator and your two hands, and they don't see most life support devices as all that new, let alone disruptive. Doctors today are born into this messy system, where gadgets and the money they fetch are woven into medical training along with medico-legal considerations, pharmaceuticals, and scientific evidence. So I decided to get the perspective of someone who's been in the system for a while. A long, long while.

There are few people more recognized in the field of emergency medicine than Dr. Ron Stewart, who is widely viewed as the grandfather of the specialty. After starting out as a family doctor in a Nova Scotia fishing village, Ron went on to essentially found emergency medicine in both Canada and the U.S., before returning to Halifax and becoming minister of health for the province of Nova Scotia.

Ron has gathered more honours than I can list, being named a "Hero of Emergency Medicine" by the American College of Emergency Physicians and an Officer of the Order of Canada, one of the highest civilian distinctions available to Canadians. He was also instrumental in the U.N. campaign to ban antipersonnel landmines. Simply put, he is a giant in my field, perhaps the biggest giant there ever was. Which is why, back in 2008, I'd been stunned when, after I landed in Halifax to speak at a local emergency medicine conference, I found Ron, dressed in an unassuming sport jacket, waiting for me at the curb outside the airport terminal in his little rust-coloured Suzuki. Dr. Stewart explained he had come to drive me to my hotel, which in my world is the equivalent of Queen Elizabeth swinging by Heathrow to whisk you into Central London. Our drive there was anything but direct. He gave me a soliloquy on Halifax history as we toured the city, zipping up and down the hilly streets of downtown.

I got the sense on that visit that Ron had in his memory the details of everything he'd ever heard or seen and, when faced with a challenge, would always seek out the most creative of solutions. So, when I decided I could use an out-of-the-box thinker to help me understand the way medical technology has changed the way doctors determine death, I rang him up. This was in 2020, and Ron was holed up away from the coronavirus in his cabin nestled in the forests of Nova Scotia's Cape Breton Island, known to tourists for its fresh lobster and gorgeous vistas along the Cabot Trail overlooking the Atlantic.

I told Ron what I was writing about and how the death dilemma was stressing me out. I told him this whole mess seemed to have started in the 1960s, when ventilators and defibrillators and CPR entered the scene. Turns out, that's when Ron entered the scene too.

After finishing medical school in 1967 at Dalhousie University, when ventilators were transitioning from experimental to standard kit and defibrillators were still big and cumbersome, Ron recalled one of the first patients he encountered just days into his independent practice. This was when new doctors were required to serve rural areas for two years, and Ron was on the northern tip of Cape Breton island, in a small town called Niels Harbour, home of a fourteen-bed cottage hospital.

"There was a farmhouse way back in the valley beyond Meat Cove, where I used to go once a week for a clinic," Ron told me. "A lady, Jessie MacAvoy, used to take care of old people when they couldn't stay home anymore."

It was the closest thing to a nursing home around, and Ron would show up in his jeep to check in on the eight elders. He even brought his own microscope to do urinalysis. "The place was immaculate," he said.

One of the residents was Annie, ninety-eight years old, with a fungating carcinoma draining from her breast. She was pale, a telltale sign of anemia, and Ron knew she needed a blood transfusion. He told Annie he'd get her into his jeep and take her to the hospital.

Ron mimicked a fragile, feminine voice: "No, Doctor, dear. We won't be doing that," she told him.

Ron was stunned. "That was the first time a patient ever looked me in the eye and said no." He didn't have a good response; he mulled it over and concluded that she was indeed right. He arranged for her family to visit, Jessie kept the wound clean, and when Annie began to feel pain, Jessie administered morphine that Ron had left in pre-dosed syringes. Annie died peacefully surrounded by her family.

"She taught me more in that place than I had learned in seven years of medical school," Ron said.

I thought about Annie and the courage it would take to push back against the revered authority of a physician back then in rural Nova Scotia. Ron hadn't asked her what she wanted; he hadn't been trained to. She told him what she wanted.

I tried applying Annie's bravery to today's death dilemma, but it didn't hold up. After all, by the time you are hooked up to machines in the ICU, it's too late for most patients to express themselves. It's left to their doctors and families to identify the line not worth crossing.

Ron didn't stay in Meat Cove for long. In medical school he'd expressed an interest in emergency medicine, and the surgeon Bob Scarf called him up one day to tell him the University of California, Los Angeles, had just launched the first academic department in emergency medicine and was looking for candidates to receive special training. Ron found a classmate to fill his rural post, loaded up his Volvo station wagon, and drove six days to Los Angeles County Hospital.

The next day he was on the admitting surgery service in a 2,300 bed hospital. He had never seen a gunshot or stab wound before, but that night he saw plenty of both. He also saw plenty of death and anguish. "It was so different from back home. The stoicism that is so typical of Nova Scotia was nowhere to be found."

Ron told me about his role later on as a coroner in Cape Breton: he once had to tell a woman that her three children, aged nine, ten, and thirteen, had all drowned in a lake after a homemade raft capsized. "She just looked at me and said, 'Thank you, Doctor.' I had never seen stoicism so bleakly before."

But in L.A., families weren't stoic. "They would wail. They would scream. They would grab you and pull you to the floor in grief. It was their own way of dealing with death."

I asked him what fifty years in emergency rooms in Halifax, Pittsburgh, Fresno, Los Angeles, and other cities had taught him about explaining to families that the end is near.

"In all of the places that I've been, there have been

cultural differences in how death is accepted. And I thought back to poor old Annie lying there with the breast carcinoma. I would say, 'We can do so much, but we will have to make a call soon about whether it is having an effect, and if it isn't, we make things comfortable.' I would tell them that. I don't ask, 'How far should we go?' because it's like saying 'Vote on this.'

"I try everything I can do to improve a situation, but if it's not working, I'll have to come back to the family and tell them it's not working and we're going to have to cease and desist. As for saying, 'Do you want this? Do you want that?' oh, that's a very dangerous road to go down.

"I'm not ever going to suggest the medical team was God — that wouldn't be a good thing — but the pendulum can swing the other way when mistrust is the standard, and I think what we are seeing there is an erosion of trust everywhere. But you know what you can do and what you can't do. But we aren't trusted."

I asked Ron if he was worried what technology would do over the next fifty years, and he laid responsibility for contending with the death dilemma before it gets worse with both doctors and patients, but mostly doctors.

"It's how we educate people coming into the profession. People who think beyond, 'Let's give a dose of this or that and hope for the best,' and who have the bigger picture in mind. I go back to Annie with her fungating tumour and think she was right and my arrogance to say 'I've decided what's best for you' was wrong."

But he also said the public needs to be realistic and to listen to their doctors when bad news is delivered. "We have been our own worst enemy here in overstating the possibilities, but we're aided in that by television and movies, the ERS and the *Houses*. So families think we can fix everything, save everyone.

"We need more communicators. Seeing doctors on the radio, in the media, honestly communicating, that gives some hope for the next fifty years. It revolves around the trust you build with the family, and it's not easy to do in emergency medicine. You must give them confidence that you know what you can do and you are competent to make those decisions. We will take all the facts into account, and we will tell you when we have exhausted our ability to change what is happening. And if it's not working, we are going to stop."

But in modern medicine, we tend not to stop; the default is to press on.

WHILE TV SHOWS DEPICT doctors arriving at brilliant responses to diagnostic challenges and jerry-rigged solutions to dramatic hospital power outages, at some point, even heroic Hollywood characters can't outrun death. While the lost pulse and flat line, with its requisite annoying monotone, often signify death on television, not everyone dies in this way; for many, their brain dies before the rest of their body.

Declaring someone brain dead is remarkably complicated, and I promise to get more into that soon. But in declaring brain death, things become quite simple, because you've established that the line between alive and dead has been officially crossed, even if blips and beeps from the cardiac monitor continue and the rhythmic hissing of the ventilator goes on.

For many ICU patients, however, brain death is out of reach; it's often the last organ to go because we're so good at using technology to keep it alive. It's the other essential parts of the body that fail, slowly, one organ at a time. There is no line in the sand; it's a gradual progression. All we know is, there's no coming back.

We call this multiorgan failure, and it often stems from an original illness affecting just one body system. In the ambulance, or ER, or ICU, health care workers mount an all-out assault to keep death at bay. We bring in the life support technology, because most of the diseases that set off this life-threatening progression can get better with time, assuming you don't die before you recover. All we have to do is keep the blood oxygen-rich and flowing, and most of the time, patients will come out of it on the other side and do just fine.

We'll put a tube in your windpipe to maintain a passageway for oxygen, which we pump into your lungs using ventilators. As many as a dozen medication pumps flow drugs into your blood vessels, which we surgically access using sixteen-centimetre tubes that penetrate the neck, chest, and groin to drip chemicals into your heart. Insulin, cortisol, adrenalin, dopamine, and medicines to keep you asleep are all fair game. Dialysis machines act as artificial kidneys, removing potassium, waste products, and excess fluid from your body. Specially concocted pablum is pumped into your body to provide nutrition, delivering lipids and amino acids and carbohydrates to your cells. A catheter in your bladder measures your urine output, and does it so precisely it's reported in millilitres per kilogram per hour. The tiniest drop, from 0.5 to 0.3 millilitres per kilogram per hour, will prompt a nurse to call a physician to come to the bedside and troubleshoot the situation.

In other words, I can take over nearly every aspect of your physiology. Most times, I win this battle against death. Organ function recovers. Laboratory results improve. Patients get better; they wake up, they walk out of the hospital, and they return to their families and friends and jobs and debts and everything else.

But then there are the times I lose. A slow decompensation, one organ at a time, into oblivion. The problem is this: there comes a point where I know I will lose, but I don't know exactly when. There won't be a return to life, but the line of death hasn't been crossed. It is a no man's land, where no person ever wants to be.

PART II

What Does It Mean to Die?

CHAPTER 4

Welcome to the Grey Zone

A LITTLE AFTER 6 a.m. on May 31, 2013, the buzz of my phone under my pillow woke me up. It was work calling, and I panicked. Was I meant to be working the day shift on helicopter 799, the medical rescue helicopter based in Toronto, not the night shift I had in my calendar?

But it wasn't a scheduler on the other end of the line. It was a manager.

"793 is missing."

Groggy, I asked, "What does that mean?"

"We think we have a crash site. Paratroopers from CFB Trenton are gonna jump at sunrise. We'll know more then. For now, we just want everyone to know."

The manager hung up, and I sat there wondering which of my friends might be dead.

That was the first fatal helicopter crash in the history of the air ambulance service in Ontario. Two pilots and two paramedics died when the Sikorsky S-76 helicopter—the same one I flew on early in my career as a flight paramedic—crashed into the woods in northern Ontario after lifting off from Moosonee to retrieve a patient along James Bay.

As it would later be reported by the safety board, the S-76 was the only one in the fleet that had yet to be equipped with ground-avoidance technology, and the leading theory is that, on the dark, moonless night, the pilots had lost their visual frame of reference and become disoriented. The phenomenon, called a "black hole," is well described in aviation. Without any external indicators for what's up and what's down, your vestibular system goes wacky. If you rely on your instincts instead of your instruments, you can fly an aircraft into the ground without ever knowing it. Pilots are trained to trust only their instruments when it comes to positioning themselves in space.

But other aviation crashes have been caused by the opposite problem: trusting instrument readings when they were in fact faulty. The crash of Air France Flight 447 in 2009 was blamed on ice crystals that obstructed airspeed measurements, leading the pilots to act on bad information and ultimately stall the Airbus A330, which crashed into the Atlantic, killing all 228 people on board.

Aviation has had to grapple with this safety paradox. Human error is by far the greatest contributor to aviation fatalities, and technology has seen crashes from human error reduce substantially, but there is a reason planes still have flight crews, and that's because human judgement can often beat the limitations of algorithms and programming. Suffice it to say, pilots today are almost cyborgs: humans aided closely and ceaselessly by technology.

Medicine, for its part, has been relatively slow to adopt technology to make care safer or more automated. Doctors — inclined to consider themselves masters of complex decision-making — are perhaps behind the times when it comes to acknowledging their own mental limitations. This may be why integrating technology in medicine has been so fraught with challenges. A pilot knows when to engage autopilot and when to take manual control, but a physician is, I think, often less flexible; if we have tech, we like to apply it, and we don't always reflect on the unforeseen implications of doing so.

Technology has also depersonalized the practice of medicine. Now, I barely need to go to the patient's bedside. (Though, as I constantly remind my residents, the answer they seek is often at the bedside, not trapped in a computer database.) I can log in, scroll through lab results, review X-ray images, enter medication orders, and do nearly everything else necessary to at least look like I'm doing my job. Often, consultants will review a patient's electronic chart from their office. They then enter their recommendations into the computer, never actually having seen the patient. While this makes work efficient, and provides everyone with access to electronic information relevant to the patient, it has also created a totally different way of going about the business of delivering health care. Many ICUs have abandoned their daily flowsheets, huge paper charts of trends and data that don't fit nicely on a screen. Computer outputs are often so dense, important facts are nearly impossible to locate. Discharge summaries, long a staple of communication between doctors, have gone from a few punchy paragraphs to fifty-page printouts that are thrown straight into the trash, so unintelligible is their format.

The death dilemma is, to some extent, a result of our often indiscriminate application of technology to prevent in the short-term a death that will ultimately come anyway, but it also stems from our failure to address the ways our dependence on technology has dehumanized the practice of medicine and the process of dying. In this chapter, I'll explore how patients have ended up tethered to machines, unable to die, as their doctors stare at computer screens far away from their bedsides.

FOR CENTURIES, A POPE'S death was confirmed in a rather ritualistic and unscientific manner. A candle flame was held up to the Holy Father's face to detect any air flowing in and out of the lungs, then a hammer was whacked against his forehead while his name was screamed. If he did not awaken, his death was announced. Hardly a sure-fire way to determine such a significant event. Still, it's a stark example of how death was defined in centuries passed: by the presence of consciousness and breath.

As doctors became more sophisticated, so too did the methods used to determine death. They began to rely on the presence or absence of a pulse, and the term *somatic death* was meant to signify cessation of heartbeats, either by palpation of the carotid artery in the neck or listening with a stethoscope for the valves opening and closing in the heart.

Yet technologies and medicines have continued to grow in sophistication, sometimes surpassing the wit of doctors and blurring the line between alive and dead. Mechanical ventilators can keep air moving in and out of lungs indefinitely; dialysis machines can filter waste out of the blood without the kidneys; drugs can mimic the hormones and chemicals produced by the brain; and the heart's cruise-control feature, called automaticity, means that a heart can beat outside the body for a number of hours so long as it receives a decent supply of oxygen.

One glaring example of how technology has disrupted time-tested means of pronouncing death is the widespread implementation of extracorporeal membrane oxygenation, or ECMO. It involves placing large tubes (think garden hoses) into veins and arteries to divert blood from the heart and lungs. The blood runs instead into a centrifuge pump, then through a membrane system that removes carbon dioxide and diffuses oxygen, then back into the body again.

Patients on ECMO don't have pulses—the centrifuge pump generates continuous rather than pulsatile flow — and aren't breathing, because the oxygenator, which is about the size of the Amazon Alexa sitting on my desk, does all the gas exchange work. Yet these patients are very much alive, sometimes sitting in bed reading the newspaper. (As an aside, many a jerk doctor or nurse has sent a medical student into an ECMO room to check for vital signs, only to watch the panicked junior, moments later, run for help. A classic ICU prank.)

All this technology makes it quite hard to actually die, but none of it gives any assurance you will recover. Every organ depends on the others; one by one, the list of organs in trouble can grow until I know the game is up. What's worse, the treatment for one failed organ often makes another worse. The medications needed to help the heart can turn the toes blue and cause them to require amputation. Diuretics used to stimulate the kidney can make you deaf. The tube in your trachea that allows a machine to push air into your lungs is a superhighway for bacteria to travel down from your mouth. It takes six, maybe seven days, and then you could have pneumonia. We add antibiotics, which are toxic to your kidney. Unable to pee, fluid builds up, overwhelming the heart. Starved of oxygen-rich blood, the brain starts to suffer. It's a vicious cycle, a game of medical roulette as we race to save each organ from our treatments for the others.

What's worse, in many hospitals each machine is "owned" by a different specialist: a nephrologist runs your dialysis, a registered dietician controls your intravenous feeds, a respiratory therapist monitors your ventilator, and a cardiologist tweaks your ECMO settings. That leaves me, the poor intensivist, to gather all the data and make sense of it, making trade-offs between different specialists to ensure each organ has a fighting chance. It sometimes feels like I'm the only one trying to consider the whole patient.

DOCTORS TEND TO THINK of death as falling into one of two categories: somatic death, which occurs when the heart has stopped and can't be restarted; and neurologic death, or brain death, which occurs when there is irreversible loss of consciousness and brain stem function, including the ability to breathe. The challenge with brain death is that sometimes a person can still look alive after death has occurred: their chest rises and falls as the ventilator moves air in and out of their body, and the beating heart keeps the body warm and lifelike, the green QRS complexes causing the monitor to beep rhythmically.

Brain death usually occurs when lack of blood flow to the brain, most often caused by swelling or bleeding in the brain, raises the pressure in the skull above the blood pressure generated by the heart. Oxygen can't get in, and hungry cells start to swell, making the problem worse. So even though the heart may be healthy and beating, and the lungs may be breathing, the patient might as well be under the guillotine.

Until the invention of the ventilator, brain dead people died quickly. Without the brain stem stimulating the diaphragm to take a breath, the heart, starved of oxygen, would stop in a few minutes, rendering a person dead in every recognizable way. But once ventilators came along about fifty years ago, doctors were, for better or worse, able to keep a body alive long after the brain was lost.

Debate about what constitutes brain death has raged ever since. One force driving the debate was a practical need: there had to be a way to determine that death had arrived so ventilators could be shut off and people laid to rest. But in parallel with the rapid development of resuscitation techniques and technologies in the 1960s was another medical advancement that added to this sense of urgency to precisely determine death while on a ventilator: solid organ transplant was quickly becoming available, and fresh organs were in high demand.

CAPE TOWN IS ONE of the most beautiful cities in the world. Set on a peninsula where the Atlantic and Indian Oceans meet, the city wraps around Table Mountain, named for its oddly flat summit, where tourists flock to watch the setting sun. I've been to Cape Town a half-dozen times, including a months-long stint in residency when I worked in the trauma and emergency ward at Khayelitsha Hospital.

My first visit to Cape Town was part of a backpacking trip across southern Africa. Known for its nightlife, coffee scene, wine tours, and surfing, the city offered plenty of attractions, but I was interested in an item far down on the TripAdvisor list, at number 67: the Heart of Cape Town Museum, located in the historic wing of Groote Schuur Hospital.

Perched against the northern base of Devil's Peak, Groote Schuur overlooks the wealthy Observatory suburb of Cape Town, where it once served white South Africans. While apartheid has ended and Groote Schuur remains a public hospital, a walk through its halls reveals it still caters mostly to the better-off and lighter-skinned inhabitants of the suburbs rather than the poorer Black people in the townships, who tend to end up seeking care at Tygerberg Hospital, the other main public teaching hospital in the Western Cape.

I wanted to visit Groote Schuur for one reason: it's where the first human heart transplant was performed, more than fifty years ago. After arriving to find the museum closed, I headed back to my hostel in the city centre to research its hours, which as it turns out, are by appointment only. Its curator, Hennie Joubert, greeted me with a smile the next day to personally walk me through the museum, which consisted mostly of original equipment and artifacts, and told me the story of the world's first human heart transplant.

On December 2, 1967, Denise Darvall and her mother were struck by a car as they crossed an intersection. Denise's mother was killed instantly. Denise, a bank clerk, was rushed to Groote Schuur's emergency department, where the hospital's senior neurosurgeon, Dr. Peter Rose-Innes, found she had a severely fractured skull. She was intubated and placed on a ventilator.

Dr. Bertie Bosman informed her father, Edward, that Denise was going to die.

While it's unclear just how injured Denise's brain was at the time, it was thought she was brain dead, though in 1967 there were no established criteria for brain death anywhere in the world.

Meanwhile, Louis Washkansky, a fifty-four-year-old grocer who had been hospitalized for months with heart failure, had been waiting to become the first ever recipient of a human heart (a few years earlier, a man died after having a chimpanzee's heart transplanted into his chest).

Surgeon Christiaan Barnard wasted no time. After training with cardiovascular surgeons in Minnesota, Barnard had returned to South Africa and begun experimenting with heart transplants. Having transplanted forty-eight dog hearts into other dogs, and after conducting South Africa's second-ever human kidney transplant the year before, Barnard was desperate to be the first in the world to transplant a human heart. At around 9 p.m. the same day Denise was admitted to hospital, Eduard was asked if his daughter's heart could be transplanted into Louis. After four minutes of consideration, he agreed, and by 1 a.m. on December 3, Barnard was in operating theatre 2B with a team of at least two dozen people, including his brother Marius, when Denise Darvall was wheeled in to have her heart cut out of her chest. Lying in the operating theatre next door was Louis Washkansky.

Six hours later, the operation was complete, and

Louis was wheeled out of theatre 2A into the recovery room with Denise's beating heart inside him.

Newspapers around the world intensely followed Louis's progress. He was interviewed by reporters, spent time with his wife, and by all accounts had nearly completely recovered from the operation when he succumbed to pneumonia.

As I learned on my tour of the museum, where wax figures in scrubs and old medical artifacts are on display in the original operating theatre where Louis's groundbreaking surgery took place, Barnard was a rather egotistical, publicity-seeking doctor who enjoyed the celebrity status he instantly achieved. By the time Louis died, Barnard had left South Africa on a speaking tour to enjoy his new-found fame.

Walking around the Heart of Cape Town Museum, you can't help but feel immense excitement. The accomplishment achieved in this place is perhaps unrivalled in medicine, and may not be rivalled for decades to come. Barnard may have been motivated by the wrong reasons, but he was a pioneer of surgery, and his fame is, I would say, well deserved.

But when Juro Wada, another transplant surgeon who, like Barnard, trained in Minnesota, made a similar transplant attempt just months later in Sapporo, Japan, public reaction could not have been more severe. After successfully transplanting the heart of a drowned twenty-four-year-old college student into a nineteen-year-old man with valvular disease, Wada was charged with manslaughter for taking a heart out of a living person, despite having determined, through similar means to Barnard, that the donor was deceased.

The charges were eventually dropped, and Wada would go on to become, according to an obituary in the *Texas Heart Institute Journal*, the best-known cardiovascular surgeon in Japan. But repeated criminal accusations plagued Japanese doctors who provided organs from brain dead patients, and Wada's legal troubles sowed fear among his peers. Organ donation and transplantation became taboo in Japan, and not a single organ was transplanted in Japan for the next thirty years.

Around the world, controversy about transplants abounded. Under what circumstances could it be okay to take organs from mechanically ventilated patients who were thought to be brain dead? Months after Barnard transplanted Denise Darvall's heart into Louis Washkansky, universities and governments began to form committees to urgently lay out the rules for removing organs from brain dead patients. The race to define death in a technology-enabled era was on.

DESPITE WHAT WAS HAPPENING in Japan, surgeons elsewhere, most often at Stanford in California and at Pitié-Salpêtrière Hospital in Paris, began transplanting human hearts, with varying success. The year after Barnard's breakthrough, over one hundred heart transplants would be performed. Less than half of these patients survived for more than three months, and by

1970 few places were still performing heart transplants. Ultimately, advances in anti-rejection medications would make heart transplantation viable again, but in the meantime the matter of how best to declare brain death was far from settled. Committees were struck to define brain death and set parameters by which organs could be acquired for transplantation.

It was the confluence of ventilators, which could keep brain dead people (and their organs) chugging along, with the sudden proliferation of transplantation techniques that forced the concept of brain death to be invented. By its very name, brain death implies an "other" death. Otherwise, we'd just call it death. This gets right down to a lot of the conflict inherent in the death dilemma: while Christiaan Bernard was hailed as a hero for transplanting Denise Duvall's heart, just weeks later Juro Wada ended up in jail for transplanting a heart.

Cultural differences are surely part of the dilemma I face every day. They appear to explain why, when faced with devastating news, some families behave like the stoic East Coast mother when Ron Stewart told her all three of her sons had drowned, while others wail and collapse to the ground, as the woman in L.A. did when Ron was training there.

I decided to go to the authority on the matter, an anthropologist named Margaret Lock. The author of *Twice Dead*, which is considered essential reading for anyone who wants to understand death as it relates to the modern era, Lock spent most of her academic career exploring the evolution of the concept of brain death, though she stopped short of investigating what we ought to do when someone isn't quite dead but is neither fully alive.

I had read her book a few years earlier, when a brain dead patient made the news in Canada and I'd wanted to get a grip on how brain death came to be a legally accepted way to die. A comprehensive thesis, her book made clear that technological advances had led to a world desperately in need of a definition of death other than a stopped heart. But it had left me with more questions than answers; brain death, at least, is death, but what of those who don't meet the rigid definition of brain death, or who are being supported with so much technology they likely never will?

Lock, who holds both British and Canadian citizenship, is professor emerita at McGill University in Montreal, After reaching out to her through her university email address, a few days later I was on the phone with the 85-year-old scholar, whose cv is 59 pages long and includes 21 books and 214 manuscripts (not to mention 364 speaking gigs).

Lock left the U.K. after graduating with a bachelors of science in 1961, lured by the Canadian government's brain drain effort, which included a free flight across the pond. She still has a strong British accent. While we only spoke on the phone, I imagine her mannerisms are very British too, so proper and formal our communications seemed to me. Or perhaps that's just how medical anthropologists talk.

Lock had a front row seat to the evolution of the concept of brain death, having completed her Ph.D. in medical anthropology at the University of California, Berkeley, which she conducted half in America and half in Japan, eventually spending time observing end-of-life cases in intensive care units in both countries before returning to Montreal to take a post as the medical anthropologist at McGill University's faculty of medicine.

She walked me through the history of brain death, starting right after Christiaan Barnard's heart transplant in 1967 first brought urgency to the issue. In the summer of 1968, Barnard summoned surgeons from around the world who, like him, were transplanting human hearts. At this meeting, a discussion arose about donors, though Barnard himself seemed little interested in talking about the individuals from whom hearts were taken.

There was consensus that "conventional" death — loss of pulse — made heart transplantation all but impossible; the lack of oxygen while the stilled heart was removed was too devastating to the organ, something that had been well established in dogs. It was then agreed upon that conventional death was really just a proxy for what was sure to follow: without oxygenated blood flowing to the brain, the nervous system would quickly die.

At this point, the discussion went a bit off the rails. An American, Dr. Denton Cooley, remarked that "alive and dead are such nebulous and vague terms, so ill-defined, that they will never be defined, since no one understands either the meaning of 'life' or 'death.' . . . We should not jeopardize the possible survival of the recipient while we are waiting around to make a decision whether the cadaver, as you call it, is dead or not," Lock wrote in her book *Twice Dead: Organ Transplants and the Reinvention of Death*.

An argument broke out over whether a donor needed to be dead or not before the heart was removed and if that heart had to have stopped for the patient to be dead. But then Barnard declared, "We are running rather short of time," and transitioned to another topic.

One month later, a committee at Harvard Medical School led by Dr. Henry Beecher published a consensus in the *Journal of the American Medical Association*. Advancing on the Cape Town deliberations, it stated that irreversible coma, as determined by senior doctors, qualified as death. Importantly, the report states, this would give those on ventilators with no hope of recovery a means to have support ended, while also permitting beating hearts to be transplanted.

Henry Beecher also noted that Pope Pius xii had said in 1957 that it was "not within the competence of the Church" to determine death (an argument I have not used with Catholic families before but that I've now put in my back pocket).

Throughout the 1970s, the Harvard criteria would be challenged in numerous court cases, and by 1981 it was clear that defining brain death was causing so much legal and medical debate that public policy was urgently needed. A special President's Commission, consisting of doctors, theologians, and philosophers, reported in July 1981 that the Harvard criteria were obsolete and stated that the focus in determining death should be on the death of the human being, not on any one organ. The language used in the report discusses the status of "the person" rather than the physical state of the body, drawing a connection between the ability to inspire and pump oxygen to the brain with the ability for the brain to be in a state of consciousness, by which a person was deemed whole.

This is where the concept of "personhood" first emerges in the debate, and it is critical to navigating the death dilemma. Mind-body dualism, as framed by philosophers like Hans Jonas, tie the meaning of life in Western society to more than the subsistence of cells. As Jonas wrote in 1974, "When the brain dies, it is as when the soul departed: what is left are 'mortal remains.' Now nobody will deny that the cerebral aspect is decisive for the human quality of life of the organism ... [but] the extracerebral body [has] its share of the identity of the person."

The Uniform Determination of Death Act was born out of the work of the President's Commission, and to this day "personhood" is a key component of death determination. But other criteria, like the irreversible function of the brain stem, which stimulates breathing, are included in the act, even though the ability to have consciousness—or personhood—rests elsewhere in the brain. So how was the personhood concept actually to be applied? Why refer both to brain stem function and personhood, if personhood is our truest definition of life?

The Death Act, which was supported by both the American Medical Association and the American Bar Association, would form the basis of similar regulations and accepted practices adopted around the world. But debate still raged. In a pluralistic society, there was no consensus that doctors had pinned down the line between alive and dead. The mind-body dualism that placed personhood in the brain was disputed in various cultural and religious circles, many of which placed the soul of a person in the heart, not the brain.

By the 1990s it was clear that the Harvard criteria, the President's Commission, and the Death Act hadn't adequately defined death in a pluralistic society. This was when Lock decided to write *Twice Dead*.

She found the essence of her inquiry very disturbing. Lock recalls seeing families torn apart over what to do when confronted with brain dead loved ones. "Certain family members would want every medical person out of the room so their loved one could die in peace, while others were attuned to the idea that this death could be made into a greater good and help others," she told me. "These dramas would act out literally around the dying person. Time and time again. The family would dither, the medical team would get frustrated, and it would be difficult to get a feel of what was going to be possible."

In Japan, she hardly ever witnessed such end-of-life strife. "Families arrived at the hospital with a decision, unified around the senior man of the family about what should be done, and they would have in mind the greater good to Japanese society," she said.

After several Japanese doctors returned from fellowships in the U.S., where they witnessed first-hand the benefits of organ transplantation, Lock describes an evolution — "it was far from a revolution," she said — whereby the popular press began to promote the benefits of donation, featuring children who needed transplants and Japanese citizens who travelled to the U.S. for heart transplants. In 1997, Japanese law was changed to allow for brain death declaration and organ transplantation, though it took nearly two years before any such procedure was performed, so engrained was the reluctance to conduct organ transplants since Dr. Wada was charged with manslaughter in 1968.

Lock retired around the time brain death definitions were being revised yet again in the late 2000s, but she continued to follow the field. I asked her what she thought of the biomedical definition of death, the loss of personhood, and if she herself would be okay being declared brain dead.

"Well, now I'm much too old, nobody wants my organs, but I certainly did think about it in the past, and I have always signed my donor card, fully and completely, without reservations." She has confidence in the modern criteria for brain death. "After having been on ward rounds where people were in persistent vegetative states or were very ill and would never be back to normal, I certainly felt strongly that I would never end up in that situation. I would allow the professionals to decide when was the time."

I asked Lock what she thought I could take from her comparisons between Japan and America over the years that might help me grapple with the death dilemma.

She surprised me with an answer that seemed to have little to do with her extensive research and many publications. "Your task today is a little easier than it was thirty years ago. Surely just about everybody will have come across this thing, one way or another, on a television show or something they've read, so your task is easier in a way."

I couldn't believe my ears. I explained about ECMO and dialysis and intravenous nutrition and how people just lingered as I built bridges to nowhere. She didn't seem to think evolving technology had much to do with it; it was the same old problem in her eyes, the problem of not accepting that death was around the corner.

"There is a bit of tension among the medical people, because they feel the families are taking too long or because the family just wouldn't make a decision. Obviously, you have to keep it that way, you can't override the wishes of the family. But you can't let them dither. Time is of the essence."

After speaking to the world expert on the anthropology of brain death and grasping the fifty-year evolution of the definition of brain death, I felt I was no further along.

I DECIDED TO GO back to Steve Berry, the death historian, to get his take on why families were so resistant to death in the modern era, why people couldn't just accept, as Steve had said, that "Pa was gonna die"?

It shouldn't have surprised me that Steve had thought quite a bit about how we've arrived at the present moment, with the death dilemma crushing the souls of doctors and families alike and damaging the therapeutic relationship both sides so desperately desire.

Steve explained to me how society is different than it was even fifty years ago. The rise of technology and loss of death as a common human experience were only partly responsible for the death dilemma. People are encouraged as never before to feel special and deserving of life, so much so that death seems unacceptable. "The map on our phone puts us in the centre of the world, and our apps have algorithms that bend reality to each individual person so that we are always right," Steve said. "Given that empowerment, every individual feels...particularly deserving of continuation of life."

This phenomenon, Steve said, goes beyond my plight in the ICU. As a teacher, he sees it too: students and parents refusing to accept his assessments of his pupils, demanding instead that he give better grades. "It's not just climate [change] denying and anti-vaxxing, we're seeing it across the board, an all-out assault on knowledge and expertise."

Steve calls it an "epistemic crisis." Society is facing a "general crisis of authority, because we all think we have more expertise than we actually do because of our smartphone. It's led to the erosion of public confidence in government, in medicine, in technology. We are in a reality war now. What you are seeing in medicine, it's happening in other knowledge sectors of the economy, where you are getting more pushback from lay people than we are used to," he said.

"We used to worship astronauts and engineers, and everybody loved American geekery, with short-sleeved shirts and pocket protectors, and all of that has been so politicized now." In other words, social media algorithms, leading the unsuspecting down rabbit holes of political spin and misinformation, have shifted society so much that individuals are emboldened to embrace alternate realities, and experts that once held authority have been disenfranchised.

Could it be that simple? Can we just blame social media and populist politicians on the disconnect between doctors and patients? I asked Steve if doctors are in part to blame for handing over our expertise to the average Joe.

"Doctors used to feel their own authority, and they used to say, 'I make the calls,' and now you're softer, you're more afraid, you're worried about the legal ramifications. People who really do know things are more trepidatious and less confident than at any time in history."

This hyped-up confidence of lay people, multiplied by the dampened confidence of those with death expertise, is only half the equation, Steve says. "At the same time, you have a deep unfamiliarity with death. It's been exotified and denied to such an extreme degree that the idea of discontinuity of the self is so harrowing to people. You also have secularization, where people don't believe in the afterlife. For a lot of folks they aren't sure about what comes after death."

I asked Steve if he could think of any way out of the death dilemma, and he gave me a quick answer: educate the masses. As a university professor, Steve loves to teach, so this answer came as no surprise, and I was skeptical, even jotting down in my notes *biased?* during our interview. But Steve was mighty convincing.

Steve teaches the course "Death: A Human History" for about thirty-five senior undergrads, and he pitched a passionate case for the career of a professor. It turns out he teaches people about death for the same reason I'm writing this book: we both feel that society has forgotten that we have to die. He told me, "What I'm hoping is that, by the end, my students will be comfortable with death, will know that it's omnipresent, and that, when death comes, I'll let go and I'll let other people go too."

STEVE HAD EVIDENCE TO back up his convictions. As it turns out, when you educate people about the end of life, they make decisions that tend to accept dying. He told me about a study done in the American Midwest in the 1990s where researchers purposely went and educated entire communities about end-of-life issues. In an area covering five zip codes in La Crosse, Wisconsin, researchers found that among 540 dead people,

85 percent had made a written directive describing how they wanted to be treated when death neared. Only 2 percent wanted aggressive intervention; the rest preferred to let death come naturally and forego invasive treatment. And this was at a time when 60 percent of all deaths in America occurred in a hospital.

I got excited when I first read the study, a few days after Steve tipped me off to it. Imagine the suffering that could be alleviated if people could be clear they didn't want to be poked and prodded in my ICU only to die anyway. But as I got into the weeds of the study methodology, my enthusiasm waned. The average age of patients in the study was eighty-two, well higher than the average age of patients in the ICU, and one-third still died in hospitals. Still, even the study's authors were surprised at how many people in La Crosse had written wishes at all, and I was surprised that most participants chose a natural death free from technological intervention.

Steve's take on this was that, when provoked to contemplate their death ahead of time, people will make measured, reasonable decisions that allow them to exercise power over how they live in the days before they die. Most people in the study didn't want to suffer or to live a life dependent on technologies like feeding pumps and ventilators.

It was clear to me that the La Crosse study was a success, and that when approached before getting sick, people are capable of making what I view as reasonable choices for themselves. Avoiding medical interventions as death nears benefits society too. Steve points to the statistics that show about a quarter of all health care dollars are spent in the last six months of life. They show, he says, that there is an economic prerogative to ensuring people know how to handle the end of life. "We get this heroic one month where we spend millions of dollars on ICU care," he said. "If we would all go a little quieter into that good night, the finances of the system would be a lot easier to bear."

I must admit, using economic arguments to justify making end-of-life decisions is awkward for any physician. But if dollars are spent indiscriminately to keep someone alive when the end game is set, and when the benefits may be outweighed by the harms and pains of technologically supported institutionalization, economics certainly factor in. I scribbled *economics* onto a sticky note and stuck it on my computer monitor. I knew that to solve the death dilemma, at some point I would have to follow the money.

I REALIZED THAT I didn't need to go back thousands of years to understand our current crisis. Steve had boiled it all down to the unprecedented rise in life expectancy since the advent of the Industrial Revolution and our new unfamiliarity with death, coupled with the burgeoning individualism of our modern day egos.

As I was processing this, Steve posed a question to me. He asked me why hospice care didn't change everything. "I always thought that the hospice movement would save us, return us to dying at home in our beds. In the Industrial Revolution, we gained many things, like the doubling of our life, but we lost a few things too, like dying in our beds. If people come home to die, and we get to see it, and be a part of it, and we become more familiar with it, then I always thought we would have a better grace, but I'm not seeing that."

It was a good point, one that's often been asked by palliative care scholars in the last few decades, and one I'll explore later in this book. But I didn't have a ready answer for Steve, other than to say that having a nice place to die doesn't really provide much reassurance to people who don't think they should die at all.

I asked Steve how he'd become a historian of death. He told me that when he was eight years old he'd read parts of J. R. R. Tolkien's story collection *The Silmarillion*. In the book's fictional world, there are elves and there are humans, and the two tribes often battle. The elves are, more or less, immortal, but the supreme being, Ilúvatar, bestows the gift of mortality to humans. This is seen as an act of compassion; allowing humans to leave the confines of the world is an expression of Ilúvatar's love for them. "If we were immortal, life would be so boring," Steve said. "There would be nothing worth doing, because there would be no reason to do it now."

Steve's eight-year-old self was struck by the idea that the ability to die was a gift from God. "You know, you look back at your life and you see stepping stones that helped you get where you are. That was a stepping stone for me."

The idea of death as a type of heavenly grace was a stepping stone for me too, and after chatting with Steve, I thought that maybe, if his course were mandatory for everyone, I wouldn't have had to write this book.

SO, WHAT WAS THE economic cost of our growing tendency to fight off death no matter what? The short answer is, it depends. In developed countries, the daily cost is approximately US$2,000 to $5,000 each day, though costs can vary wildly. But many ICUs are always full—meaning others can't always get in when they need critical care.

I decided to ask Brampton Civic Hospital, a community hospital near Toronto's international airport, where a young woman named Taquisha McKitty resided while her parents sued her doctors to keep their daughter on life support after her medical team declared her brain dead (more on McKitty's story in Chapter 5). The hospital declined to comment about the cost of McKitty's sixteen-month presence in the ICU, most of that as a dead individual being artificially fed and hydrated, so I filed a freedom-of-information request.

It turns out the hospital's twenty-four-bed ICU was at capacity 23 days in the 11 months following McKitty's declaration of death and "near capacity" for 177 days. Patients often waited more than six hours, sometimes days, in the ER before an ICU bed was available for them. Ambulances had to transfer forty-three patients who needed ICU beds to other hospitals, and four surgeries were cancelled because an ICU bed was not available.

In Canada, and many other countries with socialized medicine, the death dilemma is a matter of cost — money spent on those with no chance of survival, such as McKitty, could be better spent elsewhere, say on pediatric dentistry or prenatal assessments or public housing or a universal basic income or just about anything else that could help people live better lives. McKitty's expense to the health care system from the day after she was pronounced dead to the day her heart stopped is estimated to be about US$1.5 million.

You'd think there would be a strong financial argument to prevent cases like McKitty's from bankrupting public health care; several ICU doctors had mused to me about the costs associated with prolonging life support in brain dead patients. But not every health system faces cost constraints. In some places, these chronic, lingering patients are viewed as cash cows. In the words of one high-ranking administrator at a private U.S. hospital, "These people are indefinite revenue streams."

It didn't take long for me to find out that there were over one hundred thousand technology-dependent patients lying in long-term care facilities in the United States, pushed out of hospitals no longer willing to deal with the consequences of their treatments. Half of these patients die within a year, yet they often aren't counted in mortality statistics of top-rated surgeons and world-class hospitals because they are recorded as being "discharged." My American colleagues describe these institutions, called LTACHS (long-term acute care hospitals), as under-resourced nightmares where no sane person would ever want to be consigned. Once there, a patient was "out of sight, out of mind," one colleague told me.

Chronic critical illness in the U.S. is a twenty-five billion dollar industry. While the aging population is no doubt a large part of it, therapeutic advances that decrease ICU death rates without getting people back to health are major contributing factors. Long-term care hospitals, where ventilated patients go when the ICU doesn't want them anymore, cost Medicare over US$5.4 billion in 2014, and that doesn't include patients who require less intensive care who are sent to nursing homes and rehabilitation hospitals, which are about one-third as costly. The costs of the death dilemma are now crystal clear—both emotional and economic.

But worse than the cost of LTACHS are the realities of these warehouses. As one ethnographic study of the best and worst LTACHS in the U.S. describes, when you move from an ICU to an LTACH, the level of care you receive changes dramatically. Instead of a doctor seeing a patient on their rounds twice a day, they see them once a week. Instead of nurse-to-patient ratios of one-to-one, it's one-to-six. LTACHS are plagued by inconsistent care, weak protocols that fail to advance weaning from technology fast enough (or in some cases, are too aggressive and harm patients), less physical therapy, and overuse of medications.

What's worse is that half of all tracheostomy patients

sent to an LTACH from an ICU will die in the first year.
Or maybe that's a blessing.

I asked Jessica Zitter, a palliative care doctor who
practices in the United States but who grew up in
Canada and shares my love for socialized medicine,
about LTACHS. "They are convenient storage facilities
for things that we don't want to see. I have a huge problem with these; I talk about LTACHS a lot. People just
kick the can down the road; that's just what we do. It's
just wilful ignoring of what's really happening in front
of us. People don't understand what it means to go live
in an LTACH. If they did they wouldn't want it."

I asked her what financial incentives have to do with it.

"A lot. Welcome to the United States, Blair. It's overly
simplified to say it's all about money, but this is the problem with the United States. These chronic ICU patients
make a hospital a lot of money. Health care economics
and fee-for-service is complicated, but we've got a big
problem here."

We chatted about fee-for-service payment models,
where doctors get paid for each procedure they do:
small things like placing a central vein catheter to give
calories through an IV and big things like doing a tracheostomy surgery. Choosing *not* to do these things pays
zilch. It's a perverse incentive that doctors can't possibly
be immune to. (As a fee-for-service emergency doctor,
I know this shame all too well; I make more money
seeing another patient than I do spending extra time
to explain a diagnosis to a patient or prepare them for
discharge home.)

"Hopefully, it's gonna change," Zitter told me. "It's so out of control."

An entire new area of academia called "ICU survivorship" explores what happens to the pour souls who weren't lucky enough to die in the ICU, or as that one administrator put it, the "indefinite revenue streams" who didn't get better but didn't pass away.

The main connotation in the term ICU *survivorship* is that ICU outcomes are not binary; it's not about success versus failure or alive versus dead. For those who don't die, life may not resemble anything close to what it was before.

Declining ICU mortality seems like a matter to be celebrated. But the assumption there is that survivors return to their former lives, working high-power jobs, raising their children, vacationing on the beach, running marathons. But a 2010 study in the *Journal of the American Medical Association* found that while some elderly patients return to their baseline function after leaving the ICU, many don't.

Of all ICU survivors, only 60 percent survived longer than three years, compared to 85 percent in the general population. But that number dropped to just 40 percent if you received mechanical ventilation. In fact, if you were mechanically ventilated, you had a one-in-three chance of dying in the six months after you left the ICU, compared to one in ten for all hospitalized patients. What's more, one-third of ICU survivors ended up back in hospital within six months.

Other studies have found that ICU survivors suffer

from extreme weakness, nightmares, post-traumatic stress disorder, depression, and other psychological illnesses. Surviving an ICU admission might not be as great as is seems.

PERHAPS THE MOST EGREGIOUS aspect of the for-profit evils of the U.S. health care system was exposed by a 2018 ProPublica report that confirmed what so many ICU workers feel at top-notch U.S. medical institutions: sometimes palliative care is purposely withheld to avoid damaging statistics. In an example of how quality metrics can exacerbate perverse behaviour, solid organ transplant patients — those who receive the hearts and lungs of brain dead patients to earn a second shot at life — are deemed by federal regulators to have had successful operations if they survive for one year or, more precisely, 365 days. This has led to a phenomenon where, for an entire year, patients whose bodies have been ravaged by immune system rejection, unrecoverable infections, or layers of medical complications are encouraged to push on until they slide across the 365-day plate. On day 366, palliative care is offered and technology often withdrawn.

The ProPublica investigation, in addition to reviewing emails and texts between medical team members and interviewing hospital workers, presented audio tapes of doctors discussing keeping a sixty-one-year-old navy veteran alive until the one-year anniversary of his heart transplant surgery.

"I'm not sure this is ethical, moral, or right," said Mark Zucker, the doctor in charge of transplants at Newark Beth Israel Medical Center, but keeping the patient alive was, Zucker told colleagues at a meeting, "for the global good of the future transplant recipients." Referring to an upcoming report on transplant outcomes, Zucker was ruthless: "If he's not dead in this report, even if he's dead in the next report, it becomes an issue that moves out six more months," he said, presumably worried another death could spark an audit of the transplant program.

The federal rules have teeth. Since the rules were implemented in 2007, over twenty hospitals have lost their right to perform transplant operations. With a heart transplant being worth over a million dollars a pop (some can generate bills of over ten million dollars), that affects hospitals' bottom lines.

With such perverse and powerful reasons to keep patients alive, it's no wonder palliative care options are kept secret from many. This is not a problem at just one institution; I've spoken to ICU doctors at over a dozen of America's top university hospitals who have shared stories of transplant physicians selling families a bill of goods that at best is seen through rose-coloured lenses and at worst is plainly deceptive—a false optimism that seems so plainly unethical yet is allowed to perpetuate. In my own experience, I've been told I am not allowed to discuss prognosis or palliation with ICU patients who have received transplants, a circumstance that has, at times, led to me crying in offices of senior doctors who see it as I do but fear for their own skins as much I fear for mine. So we push on. Until day 366.

HAVING GAINED A GRASP on the shift in society where death has become regarded almost as optional, I decided to return to the world of biomedical science. Perhaps I would be on firmer ground if I could nail down a mathematical formula for death, a pure arithmetic.

I called Dr. Andrew Baker. Baker is one of the authors of Canada's guidelines for brain death. He is nothing short of a legend in the critical care universe, and as soon as I heard him on the other end of the line, I knew his was the voice you'd want to hear if terrible news was headed your way.

Baker conceded the complexity of the death dilemma yet gently and confidently held firm on what, for him, is not up for debate. "There is only one death," he said. "Death of the brain stem and the irreversible loss of [the capacity of] consciousness."

But wait. What about the Pope's breathless body, or the pulselessness I used to establish death as a paramedic?

The role the heart plays is complicated, it turns out. As Baker put it, "If your heart stops, you might not be dead. It could autoresuscitate." In other words, a stopped heart can, on its own, start beating again — although it isn't exactly common, and it must happen within minutes of flatlining. More likely, he explained, a doctor like me would intervene to restart a patient's heart and restore blood flow to the brain. Failure to restart the heart would mean the brain wouldn't get oxygenated blood. Therefore, a lack of oxygen or blood flow is simply a precursor to brain death, the "one death" Baker insists on.

This articulation of death wasn't made clear to me in medical school, or residency, or fellowship. Baker's seemingly simple "one death" construct may be clear, but it isn't how doctors are trained to think, or how the public, conditioned by movies and TV, views death. On reflection, though, I think Baker is very much right.

So what does death mean in light of organ-supporting advancements in technology? "We have to draw a line," Baker said. "A white blood cell can live outside the body for hundreds of years. We could take your DNA and insert it into a cell, and it would make protein. I can transplant your kidney into someone, and your kidney would be alive. Does that mean you are alive?"

Baker would say no. He places ultimate value on the brain above every other organ, because that's where, at least scientifically, Andrew Baker, or Blair Bigham, or you, reside. You can transplant someone else's heart or kidney or liver into me, and you'll still get Blair Bigham waking up after the anesthetic wears off. But cut out my brain and it's bye-bye.

The line, Baker believes, lies with consciousness — what he calls "personhood" — a line consistent with practice throughout Europe, the U.S., and Australia. Technology, he adds, means we must be firm in how we define death. And what that means, he says, is that when neurologic death is proven to have occurred, personhood has ended.

Personhood seems a bit jargony for my liking. I would prefer to consider it my personality, or maybe my memories, and my mom might think of it as my soul. It may mean different things to different people, but most cultures have an equivalent concept. Whether you call this intangible but unmistakable human quality the soul, the inner self, the *jiva*, the *kokoro*, the *ruh*, the *thetan*, the *nawa*, the *atma*, or the dual souls of Taoism, *hun* and *po*, you are referring to the spiritual, intellectual, personal self that makes me, me and makes you, you. Which brings us back to Baker's belief that the death of the brain is the only death that matters.

BUT DIAGNOSING BRAIN DEATH is not as easy as it may seem. There is no pulse to feel for, no electrical lines on a screen to detect. Doctors aren't flying in the dark, though. A previous lack of written documentation led experts, including Baker, to create guidelines for death determination in Canada based on rigorous science.

Written in 2006, these guidelines outline how neurological death can be declared. They are strict and, in the case of organ donation, require two physicians to verify irreversible death of the brain. The three main requirements to be considered brain dead are simple enough. First, you must have a reason to be brain dead; if doctors can't find a reasonable explanation for your state, they must keep looking. Second, you must not have any confounding factors that could be mimicking brain death: any drug that could affect the assessment must be cleared from the patient's body and, if any doubt exists, neuroimaging studies, often done with contrast dye or radioactive particles, are performed to prove that blood isn't flowing to the brain. Lastly, a detailed exam of the cranial nerves must be performed.

Despite a five-year residency and two-year fellowship, I still struggle with exam questions about brain death. The wiring of various nerves is complex, and it has never stuck in my memory very well. For example, if your pupil fails to constrict when I shine a light in it, there are at least a half-dozen locations on the nerve pathway that could be affected by a tumour, a virus, or a stroke in a brain that is very much alive. It's no wonder, then, that brain death exams are meant to be methodical and meticulous, occurring with two skilled physicians who must be in agreement. Often, a checklist is used. And having witnessed several brain death exams, I have great confidence that when an ICU doctor declares a patient brain dead, personhood has been irreversibly lost.

But there is at least one problem with using "personhood" as a proxy for being alive, or perhaps more accurately, for not being dead. And that problem is Sandra, an Argentinian orangutan (well, she's actually from Borneo, but she grew up in Argentina) who now lives in Florida.

Sandra and I are the same age; we have both been described as "inquisitive"; and we both enjoy roaming around draped in a shawl. And under the law, we are both persons.

In 2015, Argentinian judge Elena Liberatori ruled that Sandra was legally not an animal but a non-human person entitled to some legal rights enjoyed by people, including better living conditions than those provided by the Buenos Aires Zoo. The zoo couldn't provide sufficiently improved quarters for Sandra, and she was eventually sent to an orangutan sanctuary in Florida.

"With that ruling I wanted to tell society something new, that animals are sentient beings and that the first right they have is our obligation to respect them," Liberatori told the Associated Press.

While this little anecdote is a bit silly, it goes to show that the idea of personhood is far from perfect. There have even been attempts to quantify the soul. Over a century ago, Dr. Duncan MacDougall set out to measure the weight of the soul. The Massachusetts physician found that at the moment of death, a man lost twenty-one grams in weight. He hypothesized that this was the weight of the soul, and repeated the experiment in a dog, whose weight did not change, because dogs (allegedly) don't have souls.

While MacDougall's pseudo-experiment has been widely criticized, the notion that the soul has weight has persisted. The 2003 blockbuster movie *21 Grams*, starring Sean Penn and Naomi Watts, explored the meaning of the soul, and other pop culture references keep the notion that the soul can be quantified alive and well.

These diversions aside, as the line in the sand for

determining death, loss of personhood hasn't yet gained universal acceptance, and it may never be achieved.

If everyone agreed that "personhood" is the proxy for life, this book would likely end here. Well-trained doctors could tell you when someone had lost the essence of what made them human, and we could all move on with our lives until we found ourselves in a similar fate. But not everyone agrees with doctors like Baker and me, and once brain death or multi-organ failure occurs, what follows is often a courtship of sorts as doctors prepare families for the inevitable. Sometimes, those conversations are beautiful, effective, and compassionate. Other times, they lead to a disintegration of trust between the medical team and the family. In extreme cases, families abandon the medical team altogether and lawyer up. You end up in a situation where it's not clear who gets to decide if someone is alive or dead, and things get ugly.

CHAPTER 5

Declaring Death:
Who Decides When the
End Has Arrived?

You're Dead When a Doctor Says You Are

AT A CARDIOLOGY CONFERENCE a few years ago, I attended a session where a survivor of cardiac arrest was speaking. Ten years ago, you would never see a survivor at a conference, let alone giving a presentation, but having survivors speak about their experiences had come into vogue.

The speaker was a young woman with a congenital heart problem. She was on stage with her life-long cardiologist, an older man in typical cardiologist garb — sober collared shirt, perfect tie, and expensive suit. She recounted a familiar story of cardiac arrest: a lack of memory of the event, a guardian angel bystander, courageous paramedics. In the emergency room, doctors like the ones who filled the auditorium had tried to resuscitate her but had failed. They were about to quit when her cardiologist, who had somehow found out his patient was downstairs, burst into the room and said, "Keep going!"

The team rallied, and the woman regained her pulse. She would soon undergo heart-lung bypass and an eventual heart transplant, and the woman is alive today.

One of my colleagues stood up afterwards and asked the cardiologist what many of us were thinking: Why had he gone to such extreme measures, attempting to resuscitate her far beyond a reasonable time period?

"I just knew it wasn't her time yet," he said.

And, in a room full of science diehards, everyone nodded.

Whatever it is, doctors often have a fundamental ability to piece it all together. In seconds, we understand things we don't formally stop to consider, merge a thousand disparate datapoints to see patterns form, and from them piece together a coherent interpretation of what is going on in a person's body. On the surface, it's as close to magic as I can think, but at its core it's the farthest thing from it. It comes from a decade of study and seeing patient after patient after patient.

I'm sure that cardiologist, who had known his patient for years, wouldn't be able to tell you if it was the pallor of her skin or the way her ECG tracing looked or an out-of-place piece of the story that made him conclude it wasn't her time. To me, it doesn't really matter. The point is that doctors are generally pretty good at what we do, and if you trust us to do our job, we'll usually make the right call.

If only it were that simple.

SONNY DHANANI, CHIEF OF the pediatric intensive care unit at the Children's Hospital of Eastern Ontario, is one of the world's leading experts on what it means to die. From organ donation to palliating ICU patients to euthanasia, Sonny has researched how people die for two decades. As a pediatric ICU doctor, he has treated tiny babies and teenagers and everyone in between.

I wanted to know if Sonny agreed that doctors should be the ones trusted to decide when life has ended.

"In the medical context of treating disease and identifying no hope for recovery, someone has to own this. From a pragmatic stance, we can't just say families get to decide when you're dead. We can't have different religious people do that. It's not practical. The physician owns this space. Death for me is very biological. There is a definition of death, a determination of death, and a declaration of death."

I asked Sonny about the differences between countries in how they determine death; even in my own observations, there seemed to be some variation.

"There aren't catastrophic differences," he said. "Variability in determining death is consequential, though, because if we say a patient is dead but then the family sees a blip on the monitor, they can lose trust in us."

Sonny thinks that science on the last moments of life is important in helping everyone understand what dying looks like. "It builds trust if people know that the heart can start and stop at the end of life. If we find nuances in the science, we can be open and transparent about that."

This is essentially what Andrew Baker, the ICU expert who developed brain death guidelines, called "autoresuscitation." But Sonny doesn't like the term. "These people don't wake up and start breathing. They don't actually resuscitate. But their heart flicks on and off for a minute or two.

"For me, there is no dilemma around death. It's more a *dying* dilemma. There is a pendulum of paternalism. There is an era before we trained where the white male doctor in a white coat said, 'This is how it is,' and there was a lot of respect for the physician in society. We've now come to a point, aided by Google, where most of us aren't white, aren't male, don't wear white coats, and we aren't paternalistic at all. We give families choice, unfair choice. What kind of a choice is it when I say to a mom, 'Do you want to let your two-month baby girl go?' That's stupid.

"So maybe we actually need to be more fair to individuals. We need to empower people to learn as much as they can, and give them time. But we also need to support them with our own recommendations, because we have the expertise."

A lightbulb went off in my head. We were getting somewhere!

"Everything in society needs to get pushed too far one way before it normalizes," Sonny told me. "I think it's great that doctors have less control and that families have more control. But if we bring people together and give them time and transparency and knowledge, we could take more control in this. There is a consequence to patients and families when we put all the decision-making on them.

"The idea of hope is difficult. What are we hoping for? The motivations are right, because ... we have seen people turn around.... Our expertise and experience give people hope. When I see a catastrophic injury I say, 'Your job is to be hopeful, and my job is to be realistic, and we'll come out somewhere in between.' So we are to blame for hope, but that's not so wrong, especially in the beginning. Families need time to transition from hope to despair, and that's what we're not good at. We get locked in to the hope and we can't get out. That transition is where the gap is."

To improve that transition, we need time, Sonny says. He drew on recent experience: "We spent hours a day over two months with one family. It was just conversation. This family and our team, we never had conflict despite one complication after another. But it's because we put in the time."

In fact, a 2000 study in the *British Medical Journal* found that doctors tended to see the end-of-life period through rose-tinted glasses, estimating patients' remaining time to be 5.3 times longer than they actually lived.

So we do get it wrong—but in the other direction. Rather than being prone to cutting life short, we let it drag on, failing to see the forest for the trees until the last remaining good that can come from tragedy— organ donation—isn't possible anymore.

Sometimes, doctors are so compelled by hope to keep going that they can run afoul of patient wishes.

ALMA ESTABLE HAS LIVED in Ottawa since 1976. The daughter of two medical scientists, she is a social researcher. I wanted to speak with her because her father, a retired medical professor who had taught at Laval University, suffered a fall in 2016 and later on went into a coma at an Ottawa ICU. Estable told me that doctors suggested life support should be discontinued. Her father wasn't declared brain dead, but Estable says the Ottawa doctors told the family that recovery was unlikely. She adds that they asked her to designate her father a "do not resuscitate" patient and to not escalate treatments. But Estable, who shared power of attorney with a sister and brother, said no, and a bureaucratic tug-of-war ensued that drove her family and the medical team apart.

When we spoke, Estable was quick to clarify that the subsequent controversy was not about her father's death. "There was no controversy around his death," she replied sharply in answer to my first question. "There was controversy around his life." She told me that her father had clearly expressed that he wanted to be kept alive even if his quality of life was poor. The hospital, however, challenged that decision and brought the family to the Consent and Capacity Board (CCB), a quasi-judicial tribunal. When families and doctors in Ontario get stuck in a disagreement, either party can file a motion with the CCB, which sometimes mediates between patients, their families, and their health care providers. The board can appoint a representative to make decisions on behalf of patients, ruling for or against a surgery, treatment, or withdrawal of life-sustaining supports.

Estable says that the experience left her and her siblings feeling bullied. "We were constantly encouraged to change our minds. This process was as close to persistent harassment as I have ever experienced in my entire life," she said. She told me she continues to be "flabbergasted" by the pressure put upon her and her family. "It was Kafkaesque. It was so bizarre. Every mortal being leaves this world. We aren't foolish, and our father was on that path. But let him walk it himself."

As children of medical researchers, Estable and her siblings immediately scanned the literature to understand their father's condition. They used resources in the hospital to ensure his wishes were respected; doctors, nurses, social workers, ethicists, and the hospital chaplain were consulted in hopes of finding a resolution. But the hospital still turned to the CCB. Estable's family hired a lawyer and ultimately won the case at the CCB. She says her father regained consciousness and spoke with his family before he died later that year. The Ottawa hospital told me that it supports the work of the CCB and that "while we are not in [a] position to comment on the decisions of the board, their work allows cases to be analyzed through a defined, open process that hears all sides."

While Estable's father was never declared brain dead, the case is a stark illustration of the pain doctors can inflict upon a family in their attempt to advocate for their patients. It also shows how discussions at the end of life — which are often poorly broached — can disintegrate the therapeutic relationships doctors are taught to foster.

Estable has thought long and hard about her family's experience. "When can the state take a life?" she asked, not entirely rhetorically. At this remark, I couldn't help but wonder if that was how families view my role as a doctor: Am I a state actor, fancifully taking a life here or there?

Past conversations with my patients' families flashed through my mind. I felt guilty, wondering if I too had left families feeling bullied. I asked Estable what she thought should be done in the cases of the brain dead bodies being ventilated by machines while the courts debate their demise. She replied, "Why not let them be? Those families are already suffering so much." Am I cold, clinical, for wondering, wasn't that the point? Must we not suffer and grieve to move on? In accepting death, families can work through loss and suffering. Isn't my role as a doctor to communicate death clearly so that grief, then acceptance, can come in due course?

Medicine versus the Law

I'd like to think that the determination of death is firmly in my wheelhouse, that doctors and other qualified health professionals can be entrusted with the job of determining when death has occurred. (Of course, sometimes it's so obvious anyone could do it: transection, decomposition, decapitation, gross charring . . . not pleasant, but not hard to tell that death has irreversibly taken place.)

Yet doctors are often made to defend their death diagnoses in court. Many of these court cases are high profile and become case studies in health policy in the countries in which they are ultimately settled.

Other legal challenges have been brought in cases where brain death criteria hadn't been met but doctors wanted to cease life support measures they viewed as cruel and without purpose.

And of course, groups supporting and opposing euthanasia have found themselves in high courts in recent years, leading to a patchwork of law and policy around the globe regarding medically assisted deaths.

But perhaps the most surprising of these are when courts second-guess a diagnosis of brain death. As Andrew Baker explained to me in meticulous detail, medical standards around the world have more or less perfected algorithms that confirm the irreversible loss of consciousness, so how, I wondered, could two high-profile cases have been brought before Canadian courts by families challenging determinations of brain death made by doctors? The answer was painfully obvious: they weren't protesting the determination that consciousness would not return, they were questioning whether the ability to have consciousness mattered at all. It was a fight over personhood.

In September 2017, two Toronto-area families filed applications with the Ontario Superior Court to challenge doctors at two different hospitals—Brampton

Civic and Humber River—who had made declara-
tions of brain death. Both families saw initial victories,
obtaining court injunctions to force the hospitals to
maintain their loved ones on life support.

One of the patients was Taquisha McKitty, a twenty-
seven-year-old Christian woman who was declared
brain dead after a drug overdose. The other was Shalom
Ouanounou, an Orthodox Jewish man who, at twenty-
five, suffered a severe asthma attack and was declared
brain dead by his doctors. In both cases, the families
argued it was within their rights to define death in accordance with their interpretation of their religion. According
to the respective families, the final line between life and
death was marked only by cessation of a heartbeat, and
the timing of the final beat was up to God.

When I showed up with press credentials at the
Ontario Superior Court building near the Toronto Pear-
son International Airport to cover Taquisha McKitty's
case for a Canadian magazine, it was the first time I had
been in a court room, aside from the time I decided to
fight a speeding ticket (I lost). McKitty's family and their
lawyer were on one side, and the doctors and their team
of lawyers were on the other. The fact that McKitty's
family was Black and the doctors were white made
visual what was already a palpable division. I debated
which side I ought to sit on, my journalist's instincts
trying to avoid a sense of bias while my scientific brain
pulled me to the side of the doctors. I sat in the back
row of the doctors' side.

For hours, I listened to testimony from both sides.

The doctors were clear: McKitty met the well-established criteria for brain death. The family was equally clear: as long as McKitty's heart was still beating, she was alive in the eyes of her god. At one point, a projector played videos of the hospitalized young woman on the wall. McKitty's fingers twitched, and everyone in the courtroom nodded, the doctors likely seeing proof of spinal cord reflexes that had nothing to do with the brain, the family likely seeing the movement as a sign of life, a reason to hope. At that moment, it was clear to me that the courtroom was no place for this debate.

When it was time to leave, I hung out in the hallways to try to catch a word with the lawyers. That's when McKitty's mother walked towards me. I was struck by the pain evident in her face, but there was more than sadness, and more than anger. There was a hollowness, and I felt that she knew her daughter was gone. I wanted to speak to her, to hear her story, but I couldn't bring myself to do it. I turned away as she walked past me. I had a sinking feeling: if everyone in that courtroom, including McKitty's family, knew she was dead, what were we all doing here?

LEGAL CHALLENGES LIKE THE McKitty and Estable cases are not unique to Canada; court battles in the U.S., U.K., and elsewhere have gained notoriety, including the U.S. case of thirteen-year-old Jahi McMath, who in 2013 was pronounced brain dead after a tonsillectomy-gone-wrong. Jahi's family was able to raise funds to have her flown to New Jersey, known in the legal community for its protective laws in cases like hers. While religious advocates celebrated the move, medical professionals considered it desecration of a body.

The law, with few exceptions, is mostly silent on defining death, and the courts have shown great distaste when death-defining battles end up in front of judges. But that's why these cases keep ending up in court; when doctors and families resort to judges, judges fall back on outlandish delays, vague rulings, and legal mumbo-jumbo that's even worse than the mumbo-jumbo doctors use to discuss death in the first place.

Each time, rumours of hypothetical Supreme Court rulings raise panic among medical professionals. Fears are stirred up that our hands will be tied and we'll be forced to tend to hopeless sacks of cells, void of personhood, in the name of religious rights or personal liberties. Politicians are lobbied and doctors draw alarming pictures of "ventilator farms"—dead bodies being fed and watered at a cost of around a million dollars apiece each year—bringing a cold, economic face to the consequences of such a decision. Religious groups paint doctors as mad scientists in thrall to a god complex, stealing organs from the young and killing off the elderly.

With the McKitty case, experts feared chaos if the court determined families could dictate that care continue long after doctors and nurses declared it was futile, or if each individual were to define their own criteria for death.

Court rulings often mention the need for elected parliamentarians to establish laws based on societal norms, but no champions have emerged in the political arena. How this ends is anyone's guess. But it's clear that when families and doctors battle in court, no one wins.

ARTHUR CAPLAN, A WHITE-HAIRED academic who likes to answer questions with questions, seems fascinated by this topic. But the NYU Langone professor, one of the most famous bioethicists in the world, isn't sympathetic to families who want to keep patients with no hope of recovery on mechanical support.

"Buddhists believe you need to wait for the ancestors to come back in three days, but that isn't what the state says," he explains to me over the phone, his point being that modern society needs to take a position and stand with science. He adds that evangelical Christians believe in miracles and resurrection, but we don't force those beliefs on doctors and nurses applying medical standards. Technology has allowed advancements in medicine that the state must take into consideration.

Caplan tells me that five U.S. states have legislation allowing for accommodation when a family disagrees on a philosophical level with brain death. That's lead to situations where families transport loved ones who have been pronounced dead across state lines to avoid having to bury them. In those states, which all work a little differently, families have the right to a second opinion; if the diagnosis is confirmed, they may be accommodated in their belief, but "that doesn't mean the state pays," says Caplan. "It may be as simple as a hospital saying, 'Okay, you can hire nurses and an ambulance and take them wherever you want, but they aren't staying here.'" Those who can't pay get no grace from hospitals, which usually send a letter stating the time and date the machines will be turned off.

New Jersey's laws are the most lax; it's the only state that allows brain dead people to be cared for indefinitely, which is why Jahi McMath was flown there from a California hospital.

Caplan understands deeply how legal tools have been used in lieu of philosophical debates when the relationship between doctors and families moves beyond reconciliation. We chatted about the assertions lawyers arguing against brain death have made, and how those arguments most often fall flat in the U.S.

I tell Caplan that parts of the Ontario court cases argue that an accommodation for disability guaranteed by the Canadian Charter of Rights and Freedoms should compel the government to pay for ongoing artificial support. (The argument fell flat; the judge in the McKitty case ruled that, as a dead woman, she was not protected by the Charter of Rights and Freedoms.)

"You're different in Canada, because the human rights framework never comes into play here in the U.S.," Caplan told me.

I had no desire to turn this book into an essay on comparative bioethics around the world, but I still wanted to get a second opinion. I called up Kerry Bowman, a Canadian bioethicist at the University of Toronto, for a uniquely Canadian point of view.

"The boundaries between life and death are socially and culturally determined, and they are always shifting," said Bowman. "It becomes a philosophical debate."

"Descartes said, 'I think therefore I am,'" Bowman reminded me, explaining the medical point of view that Andrew Baker, the brain death expert who testified in Taquisha McKitty's trial, described as personhood. "The converse of that would be 'I don't think, therefore I am not,'" but that belief may not resonate with many religions, Bowman says.

I try to cut through to the issue of government responsibility to pay. I feel guilty bringing up cost; everyone I've spoken to has tiptoed around it, and it's time I address it head on.

"We don't really want to say it out loud, but all these people will be ventilator dependent, and there are very high costs and resources for that, and it would be part of our collective responsibility," says Bowman. An ICU bed, according to Baker, costs about $1.5 million a year to operate. "Big picture, it is part of the conversation," said Bowman. We talk about the cost of "ventilator farms" — hospitals dedicated to artificially supporting the dead with feeding tubes, dialysis machines, intravenous drugs, and ventilators — and agree that such a situation would be unlikely given how few people would actually elect for such an existence.

For that reason, Bowman sees the courts as an

appropriate, though not perfect, venue for this debate when it can't be settled more amicably at the bedside. "I think our courts are going to have to give us some direction. We need clarity." Without being a lawyer, I had read enough court rulings in these cases to know that relying on the courts was a fool's errand; the law was too vague to be applied to such messy questions. Sitting around waiting for new laws seemed equally hopeless; in the case of New Jersey, it was religious zealots who pushed for a change in law that "valued life" — directly opposing medical associations. Politicians elsewhere have been reluctant to wade into such debates, deflecting to the courts, who then deflect back to elected officials to clarify societal values by writing clearer legislation.

In the meantime, Bowman sympathizes with those on both sides of the debate as they discuss matters at the bedside. "We need to avoid power struggles. We need to be as respectful as we possibly can and explain what brain death is. If someone says, 'This is not an acceptable view of death,' we need to talk to them and listen."

A FULL FIFTEEN MONTHS after doctors had initially declared Taquisha McKitty brain dead, and more than a year since I'd seen the sad acceptance in her mother's eyes, I received an encrypted Signal text message from a source.

"She's dead."

After a judge had ruled in favour of the doctors

in June — seven months after hearing the case — the ruling had been appealed, and the doctors were forced to continue the machines and feeding pablum to keep McKitty's organs functioning. In the end, while the appeal was being considered, McKitty's heart stopped on its own.

I rushed to call my editor.

"McKitty's dead," I said.

"She's been dead for sixteenth months," said my editor.

"Yeah, but now she's dead-dead."

Medicine versus Religion

I was surprised when Mark Handelman agreed to take my call and speak to me on the record. After all, in 2017, he was one of the lawyers at Health Law Matters, the firm that represented the families of Taquisha McKitty and Shalom Ouanounou, who were suing my colleagues and questioning their competence and compassion.

Handelman is a health lawyer, has a master of science in ethics, and represents people on both sides involved in the death dilemma. He knew which side of the fence I resided on but spoke to me anyway. He didn't try to change my mind; rather, he took me into the minds of the Ouanounou family, who have deeply held Orthodox Jewish beliefs and were suing the hospital that had declared Shalom brain dead after his asthma attack.

"As there is a Jewish way of life, there is a Jewish way of death," writes Rabbi Maurice Lamm in his book

The Jewish Way in Death and Mourning. The Talmud, a collection of Jewish laws, describes recognizing death in the context of searching for survivors of a building collapse, and concludes that rescuers need only dig through rubble to find "all in whose nostrils was the breath of the spirit of life," which seems to define life as breath. In this sense, the irreversible cessation of breathing indicates death, though patients on ventilators breathe through tubes placed through the mouth, and their nostrils are left out of it.

Yet another Rabbinic approach demands that, for death to have occurred, all motion in the body must have stopped, including the heart. "Some Orthodox Jews believe that because every moment of life has infinite value, irreversible cessation of cardiac function must occur," says Handelman of Ouanounou's beliefs. While the Talmud seems concerned only with respirations, Orthodox Jews believe that a lack of breath is simply an indication of a lack of heartbeat, and that stillness of the heart itself is what defines death.

"Not all Orthodox Jews take that view," Handelman confided, explaining that when an Orthodox Jew needs help interpreting Jewish religious texts, they turn to their Rabbi, who has, it seems, final say. "Many rabbis interpret it that way. It's widespread and historic. It's not a fly-by-night definition; it's centuries old."

Still, it seemed odd that one religion could have two definitions of death, one that would permit brain death and another that would not. And in Israel the picture became even more complicated when religious law and secular law began to interact. In Israel, the 2005 Dying Patient Act does not allow for ventilators to be turned off; such an act is viewed as euthanasia and is inconsistent with Jewish societal values. Yet continuing prolonged ventilation could contribute to human suffering, which is also against Jewish societal values.

After the law was criticized for failing to integrate technological realities into religious values, a creative, if not semantic, solution was proposed. Drawing a distinction between "withholding" and "withdrawing" life support, Jewish literature permits non-interference in the natural process of dying, which should remain in the hands of God. Thus was born the idea of a ventilator timer that would have to be purposefully reset in order for the ventilator to continue working. If the timer were left to run out, the ventilator would shut off. Jewish religious law does not approach this inaction from a consequentialist aspect; thus a workaround to the law has been proposed. Withholding the ventilator becomes permissible, while withdrawing it does not.

While many countries continue to struggle to define and legislate how people die, Handelman defends an individual's right to freedom of religion as they see it. "I don't want to be on life support for myself, but I still defend [Ouanounou's] own right to his interpretation of this, and his interpretation is not based on medical benefit but on his personal religious beliefs," he said.

But could society really allow each person to interpret their own definition of death, protected by the vague religious freedoms enshrined in law? What kind of society would that lead to?

I KNEW RELIGION WOULD be part of the death dilemma equation, and Steve Berry, the historian, who wants to remind everyone on earth how to die, had reminded me of that with his reference to Tolkien's elves and humans in *The Silmarillion*. I suppose, until then, I had been putting off getting into the subject of religion, having struggled with my Christian upbringing since coming out of the closet.

I grew up in a Presbyterian household. We would go to church every Sunday, attend Friday-evening Bible class, and on Saturday mornings play basketball in a church hall, garbage bins perched on tables at either end of the court to act as nets. I was even, briefly, a choirboy, though you should not infer from that any sort of singing ability.

My father, an electrical engineer, returned to university in his forties to obtain a master of divinity degree, and shortly thereafter became a pastor at a church. My mother, who retired from her government job early after a series of amalgamations made her role redundant, found a calling as the director of a Christian charity that builds schools in Indonesia. That is to say, both of my parents were die-hard churchgoers.

I like to blame this God-fearing upbringing for my delayed realization that I was queer. I drifted from the Church once I came out, and already felt strongly secular in my adult life before my career in the medical field pushed me even further away from a belief in a higher power. Yet time and time again, religion would enter the ER and ICU as families struggled to grasp illness and death.

Steve's suggestion that mortality was a gift from man's creator compelled me to start digging into the influence of religion on views on dying. I had interviewed priests and rabbis when I was a journalist covering topics such as euthanasia and brain death, both of which appear in Canadian courts from time to time and allow freelancers to ride a brief wave of explainers and court briefs for newspapers and radio.

But now I had to go beyond a few quotes and soundbites and look deeper into the way religiosity enters into decision-making around dying in the ICU, without turning this book into a comparative analysis of the end-of-life viewpoints of world religions. Specifically, I was curious how society's drift towards secularism has impacted the experience of dying, particularly for family members of patients. After all, my patients themselves aren't able to express their own wants, unlike the people in La Crosse, Wisconsin. Similarly, their families usually haven't been able to contemplate end-of-life matters, because most people who end up in an ICU do so rather unexpectedly.

I reached out to Candi Cann, a professor of religion at Baylor University, in Waco, Texas. Since graduating from Harvard with a Ph.D., Candi has authored three books on dying in a digital world, and she studies how the dead are memorialized. I thought she might be able to tell me why so many families struggle to make end-of-life decisions when I thrust urgent questions at them in the ICU.

Candi started off our conversation by challenging me to rethink some of my deepest assumptions that hospitals are there to help patients and support families.

"People don't realize that medical culture itself is a culture," she said. "Somehow, people walk into a hospital, and they let themselves be consumed by medical culture; they abide by visiting rules and hospital definitions of who's family and who's a child and who's an adult. There are a bunch of weird cultural values that are imposed on you."

She's right, of course, but I had never thought of those rules as a culture, merely the institution's opinions. Using visiting rules as an example, Candi explained that not being able to visit a patient during the hours when nurses change shift — usually 7 a.m. and 7 p.m. — had nothing to do with patients but rather with workflow at the bedside.

Hospital chapels and chaplains were an example of the bureaucratization of religion in hospitals. "The chaplains, they operate as interreligious chaplains," she said. "That creates a flattening of religious beliefs." In other words, the organizational structure secularizes religious observance. "People walk in and they don't even think to challenge these norms, they just abide by it. I don't understand that."

Like Steve Berry, Candi believes in the hospice

model. "Hospices aim to make you feel at home," she said. "Hospitals should too."

Candi sees significant failings in the way hospitals treat patients and their families. "Why is medical culture allowed to take precedence over religious culture or other cultures that we hold dear?" she asked me rhetorically.

She argued that my quest to better define death might help medical culture but would perhaps fall short of my intended purpose of settling the death dilemma. The definition of death, she told me, is not universal; while modern medicine has a hardcore definition that is rather technical and often involves expensive testing, it is in many ways thrust upon people.

Candi has studied Catholicism in South America, Confucianism in China, and the Protestant view on death, among others. What was clear to me from our conversation is that I can't paint all religions with the same brush. Even in Christianity, death is viewed differently by Protestants and Catholics. And just within Catholicism there are several interpretations of various texts. The same can be said of Judaism, as we know, and also Islam. After a few minutes on the phone with Candi, I felt like I could write an entire book on the variety of religious views of death and dying and be no further ahead in my quest to come to grips with the death dilemma.

Candi brought up a recurring theme in my interviews with experts: the disproportionate amount of health care dollars being spent in the last months before a person's death.

"I don't want my estate to dwindle to nothing," she said. But that's exactly what happens when doctors like me keep proposing treatment after treatment, adding machines to the room to support failing organs one by one.

Candi, like Steve, thinks the answer lies in education, of doctors as well as their patients. She sees a void in the system that religious leaders can fill, offering guidance at the end of life that can normalize the dying process while doctors are trying to overcome it.

Candi speaks to this with a sense of urgency, and I feel something of her exasperation.

When COVID-19 came, she thought it would bring with it more conversations about death, particularly in the media, but she hasn't seen that happen. "The first thing I did when I started following COVID was to update my will and make sure I had beneficiaries lined up. It's amazing to me that that's not the reaction of most people. I just don't understand it. I'm shocked at how little news there is about death."

I asked Candi how she might address the death dilemma. Her response was to give some advice. "If you really love your family the way you think you do, you should do all the work ahead of time. Don't make them figure it out. It's a gift when you do the work ahead of time. You are saving them from having to do difficult work in a difficult time."

It was the Wisconsin study all over again, though Candi didn't mention it specifically. But she made clear that a cultural shift was needed, one where individuals took personal responsibility for the undeniable fact that they would die and that it was their duty to their loved ones to have a plan in place.

Candi was speaking as an academic, but she was also speaking from experience. When her own mother suffered bleeding in her brain from a cancerous tumour, Candi was ready. "We had already had the conversation. It still sucked, but I had a notarized paper. She had gone to that extent to be clear, so I was doing what she wanted."

Still, it wasn't easy. Candi's brother wasn't ready to disconnect the ventilator. "It doesn't matter," Candi told him. "It's not about you." I asked Candi to describe her brother's mindset. People, Candi said, are self-centred. They feel guilt, grief, and sadness, all of which take time to process. But for her, she and her mom had already processed these details beforehand. "This is what Mom said, so this is what Mom gets," she declared.

Candi told her brother he had a few hours to get emotionally ready. "As soon as they took her off the ventilator, she died. But it was hard for me. I felt like I was the only one who stood up for her wishes." I couldn't help but wonder what her mother's remaining time would have been like if Candi hadn't been there to stand up for her.

I asked Candi how I could help the families I meet in the ICU, the ones who say they are waiting for a sign from God.

"I live in the heart of the Bible Belt, and I'm in the thick of this," she said. "There is a tendency to think,

'God will take care of me,' and I would turn to the Gospel." I was surprised at that. Candi told me the story from the New Testament where the Devil challenges Jesus to throw himself down from a great height. If God exists, the Devil says, Jesus will surely be saved. But Jesus doesn't succumb to the Devil's taunts; he replies that he will use the tools God already gave him to stay alive.

The converse of this story is the popular anecdote about a man sitting on his roof while floodwater engulfs his house. Someone in a rowboat comes by to pick him up, as does a rescue helicopter, but the man declines the offers of assistance. "God will save me," he shouts. In fact, he drowns, and when he finds himself at the Pearly Gates, he asks God, "Why didn't you save me!" And God replies, "I sent you a rowboat and a helicopter!"

Perhaps in the ICU, Candi suggested, I could take a similar approach. As the machines in the room pile up, maybe God is sending a sign. When a doctor brings up a bad prognosis, maybe God is sending a sign. "Jesus doesn't jump off the cliff and say, 'Let's see what happens.'"

Medicine versus Medicine

I was trained at McMaster University, the home of the late David Sackett, the father of evidence-based medicine. Mac, as many call it, indoctrinates its students that an analytical brain, deeply aware of the scientific literature, can better decide a clinical course than a brain that relies on intuition and—perhaps the most pejorative term I came across during my eight years at McMaster—biological plausibility.

At Mac, decisions were made based on randomized clinical trials or, better yet, systematic reviews of clinical trials, computations that mashed the results of multiple trials together. These meta-analyses, I was taught, should guide my care plans. My wit, I was told, was just a backup. Where there was no evidence, or a lack of evidence, we would often gravitate towards doing less, or at least spending less.

When I arrived to do my fellowship at Stanford, I was coming to work at "America's Most Expensive Hospital." (Despite the tagline, made up by other fellows, Stanford is not actually the *most* expensive; it just feels that way.) At first I was rather disappointed. Trials didn't seem to matter so much, and a lack of evidence meant you could try anything that might possibly effect a cure, cost be damned.

But then I began to see the other side. Stanford attracts some of the sickest patients in America, patients unique enough that they are poorly represented in most landmark trials. Beneficial results for these unique patients, attending physicians at Stanford would remind me, can be washed out amongst the ten thousand other patients in the trials scientists so meticulously perform. I was reminded over and over again to respect the patient in front of me, to use the physiologic data on screens surrounding the head of the bed, and make individualized decisions regardless of cost rather than numbers buried in digital manuscripts.

For example, delirium is a major problem in the ICU. Patients hallucinate, pick at their tubes, and holler into the air. It's as disturbing to watch as it is annoying to work around. Study after study, all of them with some heavy limitations, have shown that medications do little to reduce the time delirious patients spend in an ICU, and so at McMaster we would use them sparingly. But at Stanford, a lack of high-quality evidence gave permission to try all sorts of pharmacologic cocktails that might provide even the slightest relief from the grip of delirium. Smart psychiatrists would leave a list of up to half a dozen drugs to block or upregulate various neuroreceptors. These combinations of therapeutics could change every time a different psychiatrist came on service.

A psychiatry recommendation to the ICU team for an eighty-four-year-old delirious patient:

Please discontinue quetiapine and avoid other antipsychotics due to dopaminergic effects. We recommend starting hydroxyzine; the sedative properties of hydroxyzine are superior for agitation.

Then the next day:

Please stop using hydroxyzine as anticholinergic medications can cause paradoxical agitation in the elderly. We suggest trying antipsychotics such as quetiapine or haloperidol instead.

And according to the Society of Critical Care Medicine agitation guideline I was taught at McMaster:

> The panel recommends using multicomponent, nonpharmacologic interventions to reduce modifiable factors for delirium in the ICU. Medications, including antipsychotics, are not recommended as a routine strategy to either prevent or treat delirium.

It was up to me to hit up the medical literature and arbitrate between these "stylistic" differences and many other "stylistic" differences common at Stanford.

I THOUGHT THESE TWO divergent philosophies couldn't possibly co-exist, and for many months resisted the Stanford way. But after a while I began to realize that both these approaches could be taken simultaneously; a gut instinct based on the patient before me could be crossed-checked with a deeper dive into the minutiae of the literature to decide the best course of action, which would most often, but not always, align with the trials and meta-analyses.

Quickly, I began to test out the recommendations of the Stanford attending physicians, building some of them into my own practice while leaving a few at the side of the road, knowing I'd be ridiculed in Canada for trying such unproven, if not irrational, treatments.

But I couldn't reconcile one of the greatest differences between Stanford and McMaster: the attitude that piled more and more machines into a patient's room while their spirit and life seemed to evaporate further with each passing day. (Of course, at Mac, we would throw the kitchen sink at people who had a chance.)

While a disregard for the costs of health care allowed me the thrill of prescribing vastly expensive medications, unencumbered by questioning pharmacists and finger-wagging bean counters, I never quite got comfortable with the liberal use of some surgical technologies, such as decompressive craniectomies, where a large part of the skull is removed; tracheostomy, where a tube is cut into the front of the throat near the Adam's apple so a ventilator can provide artificial breaths; and ECMO, where large hoses are placed into arteries and veins so blood can be siphoned out, oxygenated, and pumped back in when the lungs or heart are incapable of their usual duties.

We have all of these technologies available to us in Canada too, but we are much more selective — perhaps sometimes too selective — about who should receive them. Yet I was never that uncomfortable with Stanford's willingness to *try*. Sure, the U.S. system doesn't even attempt to provide great care to all of its people, and the Canadian ethos is strongly attached to the idea of equitable health care for all (though we don't come even close to achieving this ideal), but I know how privileged I was to get in the door at Stanford; there was something remarkable about being unleashed from the constant pressure to be a steward of precious health care resources in Canada, being allowed to go in guns blazing, to use every tool in the medical arsenal. It was liberating.

But where I really felt troubled was in the decision to *keep going* once I thought it was clear the technologies hadn't achieved what we had hoped. And I wasn't the only one. A common theme, whether in Canada or the United States (or in my experiences working in ICUS around the world, for that matter), is the tension between two camps of doctors: ones who see futility and want to focus on comfort, and ones who want to keep going because they can discern a narrow path to victory by dissecting biochemical changes that can optimistically indicate improvement.

These two camps are in constant battle, in tense phone calls and hurried conversations in hospital hallways, and it's one of the most politically fraught situations I find myself in. There are some hospitals — famously "world's best" kind of places, I'll add — where palliative care doctors are forbidden from consulting on surgical patients, where intensivists can't discuss end-of-life care without other doctors coming on board. These struggles have been well documented, though we rarely speak about them. More than a few times I have suggested a palliative care consult, only to be told sympathetically, "It's a Doctor X patient. Don't even think about it!"

The topic is so controversial, it's not easy to find an insider's account to illustrate the gravity of this aversion to declaring a patient's cure unattainable. Which is why I was relieved to come across Jessica Zitter, who earlier taught us about the detriment of long-term care hospitals.

Zitter is both a palliative care doctor and an intensivist in Oakland, California. "I straddle both worlds," she told me. Zitter is the author of *Extreme Measures*, a confessional of sorts that details her own struggles with the death dilemma as an ICU doctor that eventually pushed her to become a palliative care doctor too.

I asked her how she navigates the death dilemma when faced with doctors — usually surgeons — who aren't open to the idea of withdrawing life support. "It's hard," she said sympathetically. "I know surgeons. I know this dynamic."

She lamented about the surgeons who get territorial when they feel she's stepping on their turf. "Who owns the patient?" she said. "Surgeons fire us from cases all the time. If they find that a nurse has asked palliative care to see the patient, they get angry and act like they have some right to be territorial over a person. It's crazy. But it's a lot for me to ask a young trainee to say, 'No . . . I think a palliative consult would be helpful.' It's very hard to stand up to authority — one of the hardest and most stressful things of my career. But for every ten times you do it, one time you might change their mind."

Zitter thinks the solution can't come from trainees like me; we don't have the agency and are too vulnerable. "It's easy to say stand up for your principles even when it's against someone who is from a different system of thinking than you are, but it's not fair to ask trainees to do that. It's hard for me to do that, and I've been an attending for twenty years."

She thinks striking a tone that values the principles of general humanism has to come from the top. "The chief medical officer has to make it clear that palliative care is valued and that each surgeon needs to be practising goal-concordant care. (Goals, of course, can change as complications rack up and hope dims.) The metrics that are being valued for a subspecialty practice are set from above, and you can select metrics that measure palliative care and humanism," she told me. Surgeons could be measured on, say, the proportion of patients who receive palliative care consultations, or electronic records could be monitored for completion of goals of care discussions.

And the outliers?

"Boot 'em!"

AT THIS POINT YOU might wonder why anyone would want to be an ICU doctor at all. With all this death and conflict, why bother?

Of course, the death dilemma is about what happens when ICU care fails to achieve our hopes for a speedy and complete recovery. But many patients do improve, some fully, and that's where the tension lies—we aren't always good at knowing which way the cards will fall.

There are a few subgroups of cardiac arrest patients who die 100 percent of the time, but one of them is especially dismaying: the people whose hearts are resistant to defibrillator shocks. Most people who are in ventricular fibrillation—a chaotic jumbling of electrical signals that prevents the heart muscle from pumping blood—can be defibrillated into a normal heart rhythm. But some people's hearts just won't respond. People in shock-resistant ventricular fibrillation usually have had massive heart attacks; blood vessels feeding the sensitive muscles in the ventricles get clogged, and oxygen can't reach the tissues. As a paramedic, I would shock these people over and over and over again, rushing them to an ER, where even more shocks would be given. Eventually, the amplitude of the fibrillation, the oscillating lines on the electrocardiogram, would dampen, becoming smaller and smaller until only a flat line remained. I've pronounced about a dozen people with shock-resistant VF dead, despite heroic hour-long efforts to save their life.

In recent years, we've gotten so desperate to defibrillate these people that some doctors apply two defibrillators, double-zapping the patient with some success. Some doctors will inject the medical version of Drano, a strong "thrombolytic" that breaks up blood clots, but this trick too is rarely effective. In some places, doctors hook the patient up to a CPR robot that pounds a piston onto their sternum one hundred times a minute while a cardiologist injects dye into the heart to find the obstructed vessel, then deploys balloons and stents to open it back up. Remarkably, once blood flow is restored, the hearts begin beating, albeit very weakly, but more often than not the brain is pooched—dead from a lack of oxygen.

In Minneapolis, your chance of survival is much higher than in Toronto. In Minneapolis, the odds of pulling through and fully recovering are fifty-fifty. That's because thought leaders there didn't want to give up on shock-resistant hearts. Over a decade, they built expertise and perfected their system so that paramedics equipped with CPR robots raced patients not to an emergency department but to a cardiology catheterization suite, where they were crashed onto an ECMO pump that takes over from the heart and their arteries are unclogged.

This type of endeavour is daunting. Nowhere else in America does it like Minneapolis. But it works; the survivors would have been dead had their cardiac arrest occurred in Milwaukee or Iowa City or Spokane. By pushing the envelope, the pioneers in Minneapolis upended the resuscitation community.

Medicine is an industry based on pioneering efforts. Whether with Barnard's heart transplant or the Mark ventilator or Knickerbocker's dog, it has been through attempting the unthinkable and refining it that we have gotten to where we are today. The medical community, guided by pioneers of the past, wants to keep trying to advance technology to do good, accepting the bad that inevitably comes from slugging towards progress.

So while it's easy for me to criticize my own profession's inability to just let go and allow people a comfortable death, to deny us the chance to push the envelope is to condemn medical care to the status quo. Reflecting on this makes me incredibly uncomfortable;

to get good at something, as they are doing in Minneapolis, there must be sacrificial lambs. Whether by special design, such as in clinical trials, or by the natural means doctors practice medicine, playing it safe isn't how we've been raised. We must aspire to be better, to save more lives in the future.

And that means technological advancement.

Lazarus Syndrome: Can Doctors Get It Wrong?

Flying from Toronto to San Francisco one time — or maybe it was San Francisco to Toronto (I did the trip over thirty times during my ICU fellowship at Stanford to see my Toronto-based fiancé) — I decided to numb my mind with Air Canada's in-flight entertainment options. *The Resident*, a medical drama starring a hot-shot medical trainee who finds himself in all sorts of medical catch-22s, jumped out amongst the tired selections. Ever since ER wrapped up in 2009, I've struggled to find a medical TV show that resonated; *The Resident* was the closest I'd come to the archetypal medical drama of my youth that quite likely contributed to my desire to work in emergency settings.

The titular character, Conrad Hawkins, played by the actor Matt Czuchry, finds himself at the bed of a patient his intern has pronounced dead. Zipped into a black body bag, the patient suddenly sits bolt upright, a supposed failure of the intern to diagnose death correctly. The intern is eventually exonerated, and a case of Lazarus syndrome is diagnosed. It made for great television, particularly at thirty-six thousand feet, but it also made me wonder if Lazarus syndrome actually existed.

I called up Sonny Dhanani, the pediatric ICU doctor who studies how people die, to ask him a question I didn't really want to ask but couldn't really avoid. Can doctors screw up death diagnoses?

Sonny explained that Lazarus syndrome, a pop culture favourite of medical dramas, occurs when CPR is stopped and a patient is left for dead only to reanimate a few minutes later. Case studies show that this can happen in the minutes following the stoppage of CPR — twenty minutes is the longest out that's ever been reported.

"There are a number of very good explanations for that," Sonny told me.

Often, the chest is hyperinflated by artificial respiration, which reduces blood flowing back to the heart. When you stop overbreathing for someone, they may experience some increased blood flow to the heart. Other times, they were hyperventilated and became alkalotic, which can lower blood pressure. Other times, the pounding on the rib cage stuns the heart; once compressions are held, the heart can bounce back. "So what this means," Sonny said, "is that we should wait a few minutes before declaring death."

Sonny has conducted the largest study in the world on people as they die. His team watched six hundred ICU patients die, precisely because they wanted to prove that dead was, well, dead. What they found fascinated me. It turns out that sometimes cardiac activity doesn't just stop. You don't just flatline. One in six cases found that after you flatline, you'll have a few more blips on the ECG. Sometimes, that meant patients would have an arterial pulse stop and then start again. But it always stopped once more. None of 15 percent of people who had a return of cardiac activity lived for more than a few minutes (4 minutes and 20 seconds, to be precise).

"Once the heart stops, there is no coming back, unless people intervene with resuscitation. If we want to biomedically determine death for everyone, this is how we can do it."

Sonny made clear that I had to separate the idea of Lazarus syndrome — which occurs only after CPR was administered — from the types of deaths that lead to organ donation, where life support is removed and doctors wait for the heart to stop.

The patients who autoresuscitate die within minutes, while those with Lazarus syndrome could theoretically recover. Sonny's research found only 13 cases out of 631 patients had transient resumption of cardiac activity, but none of them took a breath or regained consciousness. "The blips only lasted for a minute or two. The idea that you go down to the morgue and find someone alive, that's never been proven."

So the medical dramas that feature patients who have been pronounced dead then miraculously wake up are stretching the facts. Whew.

THERE IS NO LACK of debate between the doctors promoting science and the families wanting to make decisions guided by their religion, and I see no compromise between the two sides or, indeed, any sign they will ever agree on how the death dilemma might be resolved. Certainly, legal scholars haven't been able to bridge the divide, and doctors and hospitals, caught up in their own reputations and focused either on making more money or spending less, seemed incapable of bringing about a timely solution.

Nevertheless, after living for some time with the thoughts I've discussed in these chapters, I felt I was finally getting close to pinpointing the nub of the death dilemma. I took all my notebooks, interview transcripts, research papers, and death-related paperbacks into my living room and started to construct a thesis of why doctors like me worry we're not letting people die fast enough.

CHAPTER 6

The Root of the Death Dilemma: An Equation

THE DEATH DILEMMA WAS looking increasingly like a philosophical problem to me rather than a scientific one. Both doctors and those they were trying to serve had deeply rooted fears that interacted with technology to allow the problem to propagate. How could we bridge the divide between well-intentioned doctors spewing medical jargon and overwhelmed, devastated families clinging to hope and faith without us resorting to underequipped judges who always seemed to dodge the question?

Our innate desire to live as long as possible has driven remarkable advances in medicine and technology over the past century and led to the increase in ICU survivorship we see today, an undoubtedly good thing for many. Society has embraced this evolution, growing accustomed to medical miracles, becoming

143

enamoured by good-news stories and getting hooked on medical dramas. Yet for some, survivorship is not accompanied by commensurate increases in quality of life. The unintended but very clear consequences of this phenomenon I call "resuscitation glorification" seem to have created a societal belief that death is never near, if it comes at all, and that survival is always better than death, a position many in the know dispute.

Our collective refusal to recognize that death is ever near — a second phenomenon I'll call "death denialism" — means that we push forward with our application of medical technology. This cognitive bias, a combination of sunk-cost bias, where our prior investment in something promotes ongoing investment, and a new bias I'll call "micro-improvement" bias, where small changes in biochemistry somehow give us an unfair hope for the state of the body as a whole, leaves health care professionals, patients, and families with a misguided optimism that things are somehow getting better when the overall prognosis remains dismal.

When technology, resuscitation glorification, and death denialism are added together, the result is a rosy assessment that couldn't be further from the truth, a false hope that denies us the chance to weigh the cons of pushing on, suffering on a road leading to nowhere.

The Death Dilemma Equation:

Technology

×

(Resuscitation Glorification + Death Denialism)

=

False Hope

False hope drives us to push on in the face of dismal odds. It means that we set aside one of the most important tools in medicine, palliative care, until, I would argue, the window for effective palliative measures has mostly closed and it is too late to undo extraordinary suffering.

I have already discussed at length the life support technology that is a precondition for the death dilemma. The roots of resuscitation glorification and death denialism have also begun to come into focus. In this chapter, I'll dig into how hopes and fears allow micro-improvement bias to delay our deaths without improving our lives.

Jessica Zitter calls this the "ICU roller coaster." Once you get on it by accepting technological life support, you get tossed around, slowly getting better with micro-improvements, quickly getting worse when hit with complications, never really knowing which twist or turn will come next and having almost no control over when the experience will end.

For doctors, a fear of failure is about more than letting down our patients and their families. It's about our own sense of self-worth, our egos, and the very construct we build that allows us to endure the difficult moments that doctors face every day. For families, a fear of death comes not only from a fear of loss but also from an aversion to making the tough decisions technology has forced us to make for each other.

These fears have paralyzed the players who are most able to affect the death dilemma equation.

A Fear of Failure

If you asked any resident assigned to the overnight shift in the ICU what their job was, I bet nine out of ten would say, "Do everything necessary to keep 'em alive till morning."

Most residents rotate through the ICU one month at a time, spending maybe only two or three months in their four- or five-year residency managing the sickest of the sick. Since few residents will choose ICU as a subspecialty, most aren't overly keen to develop critical care expertise aside from what is absolutely required to survive the rotation.

Most of my friends dreaded ICU overnights; the attending physicians go home, and while they are theoretically available by phone for emergencies, every resident knows that phone calls at 3 a.m. are not well received. After all, the attending will be back at 7 a.m. for a full day of work. The unwritten rule of the ICU is just to get through the night and let the day team sort out the mess.

The same can be said for most specialties: we are there to help people, to make them better, to save their lives. Thrown from their hematology clinic or plastic surgery theatre to the ICU for a month, residents struggle to learn the medications, procedures, and machines that are "core ICU competencies." So the idea of not using some of the fanciest tools in the hospital doesn't really come up, reinforcing the "keep 'em alive" mentality.

But one ICU attending physician made clear to me that there were some patients who were destined to die and that throwing the kitchen sink at them was doing them a grave disservice. It was during my second week in the ICU as a medical student. After the gruff but friendly attending who let me perform my first intubation left the service, I ended up with a new attending known for being a grouch. He was curt, dismissive, and never made eye contact. Only rarely did he contribute something verbal on ICU rounds. On the first day he was on service, we were discussing a hopeless case of an old man whose lab panel was entirely lit up in red numbers indicating abnormalities. He was on "maximum" doses of infusions to maintain his blood pressure, and the ventilator was having trouble clearing enough carbon dioxide from his lungs.

As the team debated how to turn things around— maybe some sodium bicarbonate, we thought, or a change of antibiotics—he yelled, "Enough! We're done here. No more!"

We fell into a stunned silence. The family had asked us to "do everything," and even though none of us thought it would help, doing "everything" was what we were trained to do. But what came next was even

more surprising: the boss pointed to a bed across the
unit occupied by a similarly sick patient and said boldly,
"And he's next!"

I suspect many might cringe reading those words
from an attending intensivist. It sounds like a cruel disregard for life and an awful abruptness in handling a
sensitive matter. I thought so too, and it really upset me.
But over the years, as I replay that traumatic experience
over and over in my mind, I am less upset at—even a
little admiring of—the jerk who nearly had me abandon medicine so early on.

I now see what I believe was wisdom from his forty
years of caring for the dying, bravery in being able to
call it, and humility in being able to admit that with all
of our drugs and machines and tests, we were unable
to save these people, that anything other than a swift
passage amounted to the real cruelty.

A Fear of Death

While physicians' fear of failure can be criticized,
modified, and perhaps reframed into something more
patient-centric, there is a much harder fear to address:
a fear of death.

Doctors are often as afraid of death as our patients
are—afraid because we are taught that with death
comes failure. Death is a challenge to our professional
identity. It cuts us deeply, personally. And so we find
great relief when families tell us to do everything,
because it gives us something to do.

For surgeons and transplant doctors, it's a matter of statistics. Sure, these skilled doctors want what's best for their patients, but the system is stacked to pervert their good nature by incentivizing non-death, under the assumption that death is the only bad outcome one can experience after surgery.

For everyone else, the drive to survive is hardwired into our brains. Originating in our amygdala, a prehistoric part of the brain shared by birds, reptiles, and even bugs, it's responsible for the urge to find sustenance, to fight off attackers or flee from their grasp, and to procreate—and it means that giving in to an impending death is not something that comes naturally.

If we start to die, say when we hemorrhage blood after a table saw accident, our amygdala kicks in. The rest of the body starts to respond too: hormones increase heart rate and blood pressure. If our ancestors were being chased by sabre-toothed tigers, blood would divert from their intestines to their muscles to help them fight off the threat or run away as fast as possible. If your life is in danger, expect your body to automatically and dramatically react.

But in giving in to our primordial instinct to stay alive—to ask doctors like me to "do everything" to save you—we do ourselves a grand disservice. In delaying death, we may only cause more pain, more suffering, more despair.

Doctors and nurses know that dying is scary. We see it all the time. Patients plead with us, "Save me," "It's not my time," "I'm not ready to die," "Please do everything." And when patients can't speak for themselves, families usually make the assumption that their loved one wouldn't want to die (which, before they became critically ill, was probably true). When faced with the odds of a fate many view as worse than death, wanting to live isn't always so obvious. But sometimes it doesn't matter what we want. We can only do so much, limited by science, technology, and Mother Nature as we ultimately are.

Sometimes, we can do something, but we shouldn't. And that, I suppose, is what the death dilemma is all about. It takes wisdom to know when adding medical therapies helps and when it hurts.

WHEN I WAS TRAINING to be a flight paramedic, my preceptor, Jonathan Lee, loved to quiz me. He'd ask random questions that amounted to medical trivia, like how long does a red blood cell live, which no paramedic has ever thought about ever. One night, while flying in our Sikorsky S-76 twin engine helicopter, he asked why I had given midazolam, a drug similar to Valium, to our patient.

"As a benzodiazepine, midazolam potentiates GABA receptors, opens chloride channels, and inhibits neurotransmission," I said. Jon looked at me and said, "No, Blair, you gave it because it's a sedative and the patient was agitated." This type of thinking he called "3 a.m. thinking" — simple summaries that could be executed and understood by the exhausted, hungry, stressed brain. Jon wanted me to develop 3 a.m. models to make sure I didn't forget something vitally important or make a critical error. "You can't be a textbook at 3 a.m.," he told me. "Think bullet points, not paragraphs."

This framework has served me well, and likely helped me save lives when I wasn't at my mental peak. I decided to apply it to the death dilemma as an exercise in summarizing the gist of it, and after a few days something came to mind. Fruit.

A child walks up to four experts, each a master of one of the human senses. She asks them, "What is this fruit?"

The first adjusts his spectacles and examines the fruit. "This is yellow!" he says.

The second bends close and sniffs deeply. "This is citrus!"

The third feels it with his fingers, caressing the peel. "This is waxy!"

The fourth bites into it and scrunches her face. "This is sour!"

Yet none of them know it's a lemon. And in just the same way, well-intended medical specialists are so focused on components of the body, they forget to see the human, the person, as a whole. This tunnel vision is multifactorial. It is because doctors are trained to look at things they can fix, establishing a self-esteem system based on being able to make things better. It is because we are trained to be objective, secular, and unemotional. And it is because we are gutless, too often unable to call it, even when it is crystal clear.

But it takes two to tango.

Families often see what they want to see in their dying loved ones, focusing only on the parts of the picture they feel they can deal with. Because of faith, hope, or blind love, they take the hints doctors give them about what is to come and compartmentalize them. It's human nature.

Death Speak

Is the solution to the death dilemma simply that we need to choose our words more carefully? Can workshops and scripts save us from the agony of broken relationships between health care workers and the families they try to support?

That certainly seemed to be a common theme in my own medical training. In courses, workshops, and simulations, I've been told that if only I could listen better to patients' families, skillfully elicit their hopes and dreams and values, and adopt a firm but compassionate communication style to convey delicate information, they would see my point that a technologically assisted life — a quasi-life? — is worse than a natural death.

This hope is well established in scientific literature, which is inundated with studies of communication techniques that claim to address the death dilemma head on. But in real life, the problem persists, and I couldn't accept that it was just from a failure to translate that knowledge into bedside practice.

I was skeptical that we could talk our way out of the death dilemma — very skeptical. I sought some advice from Brian Carpenter, a professor of psychological and brain sciences at Washington University in St. Louis. Since his days as a geriatric psychologist, Carpenter has been studying the process of breaking bad news at the end of life, and I wanted to ask him if the death dilemma was exacerbated by doctors like me who just weren't wording things properly.

"There comes a point where you can't avoid the inevitable, and no matter how great the technology is, it's not going to allow people to restore themselves to the kind of life that brought meaning and purpose to them when they were healthier," he told me.

I nodded along as I listened. So far so good. He seemed to be on my side.

But when a patient's doctors can call on so much technology, he explained, the challenge for the patient is coming to grips with the fact that they're not going to have the same kind of life they had before. He started talking about some low-hanging fruit, like encouraging people to have conversations about their "goals of care," a bureaucratic term used daily in hospitals to discuss what a patient's wishes are. Goals of care are often framed as a spectrum of therapeutic options, but for most hospital-based doctors, they are pragmatically seen as either going for it—using whatever technology, surgery, medications, and so on that might prolong the patient's life—or avoiding these "aggressive" measures, choosing instead to keep the patient comfortable for whatever time they have left. (Palliative care doctors would have a heart attack reading this paragraph, but despite their best efforts to educate the masses, most doctors don't hold nuanced views about goals of care.)

"It's important to start having goals of care conversations early in the illness trajectory. That's why palliative care is trying to get their foot in the door at the moment of diagnosis so they can start to have goals of care conversations ideally before [patients] end up hooked up to all that technology and withdrawing it is much more difficult."

But having early goals of care discussions, while seemingly a good way to ease the death dilemma, is impractical at best. Even after the outstanding success of the Wisconsin study in La Crosse, which proved that precontemplating one's death meant dying better, fewer than 20 percent of North Americans have written directives to guide doctors caring for them when they are critically ill. Saying that people should precontemplate their death and have these discussions early is like saying you should line up a funeral home before you die — most people don't, and they leave it to their family to sort out when the time comes.

I asked Carpenter what I can do in the ER or ICU when a patient hasn't already thought about the kind of care they'd want to receive. When things are more sudden, Carpenter explained, you have to respect the process people go through to get psychologically ready to make a decision.

"Forcing them to make a decision before they are emotionally capable of making that decision isn't going to go anywhere. What you have to do is meet the person where they're at, but also be very candid from the medical point of view and the chances of further treatment being successful."

Carpenter spoke of another low-hanging fruit: teaching doctors how to have these conversations. "The best you can probably do to educate clinicians is to let them know that there is a process and you can't rush that process. Everyone will make their way along that process on their own timeline. For some people it might be two days, for some people it might be ten days, so the best thing we can do is to educate that this is a process."

I asked Carpenter how ICU doctors can help move the process along; hanging in the balance, after all, is a dying person tethered to machines undergoing painful procedures.

"You can plant some seeds and offer some comments and information and perspective based on your professional expertise and experience about what you think might happen, but you have to let those seeds grow at a pace the person can tolerate."

Carpenter gave me permission to plant these seeds firmly. "You must lay out the truth in a way that is clear so that there is no room for misinterpretation. State very clearly the prognosis. Being honest is difficult and painful for everyone involved, but if there isn't honesty from the get-go, you open up so many complications and possibility for things to go wrong. You don't have to give anybody false hope. Family members will latch on to that, so you run the risk of contradicting yourself."

But he also encouraged a focus on the social side of the conversation, suggesting I put less emphasis on the medical circumstances. I lamented that families didn't seem to understand the significance of the information I relay about the certainty of death: rising lactate levels, worsening acidosis, critically low oxygen saturations. I asked him what I could do to demonstrate more clearly the futility and finality of what I was witnessing so that families could decide more quickly to pull the plug.

"The numbers are useful," he said, "but it's not always about the data or the science. That's not often where people's heads are at. By slowing things down, physicians can have more holistic conversations and focus less on the technology and science of it all."

Carpenter recited tips I've heard time and again in workshops that teach how to break bad news. Things like keeping in mind that people might not be able to take in a lot of information when they are really emotional, so providing small bits of details at a time, and asking them to repeat it back to you to make sure they got it the way you meant them to hear it. I've tried all of these tips, and while they are no doubt helpful, they only go so far.

Carpenter admitted that communication skills won't always work. "No matter how skilled the physician may be at communicating, the reality is there are some situations where you aren't going to convince them, and the ethics board is going to weight in and you'll get legal wrangling. But you try to build a relationship first. That's helpful—but not always possible."

There are differences across medical specialties in how willing people are to deliver bad news, Carpenter said. "Ten years ago, oncologists were the worst. But they've really changed their approach, and now oncologists are most skillful at breaking bad news. But some other specialties, where the focus is on survival and cure and keeping people alive, they just don't have those conversations."

I asked him how the oncologists changed their tune.

"There was a very intentional effort to pay attention to outcomes. When you're not up front, not honest with people, it leads to worse outcomes. Worse quality of life, worse quality of death, more family dissatisfaction, more lawsuits, higher cost, all sorts of bad things cascade from bad communication. The oncologists didn't figure this out all by themselves; the practice of oncology became more of an interprofessional enterprise, with social work and nurses and palliative care making some inroads to help them do their job."

For many specialties, though, the palliative care conversation is a non-starter. No amount of workshops and simulations will make doctors better communicators of end-of-life matters if they themselves aren't ready to change. Many surgeons consider a move to involve palliative care experts as "giving up," and in many ways it is. But it isn't giving up on the patient; it's giving up on a curative intent and on fighting a reality that can't be avoided. It's an acknowledgement that we aren't always able to achieve what we set out to do.

The Elephant in the Room

Talking more will get us places. But I worry that a request so simple as better communication between doctors and families belies the urgency of the death dilemma; it is no secret that poor communication is endemic in the high-stress environments where high-stakes conversations must occur, and many a tool has been developed to coach doctors through these difficult conversations. I should know; I have taken at least half a dozen workshops to hone my end-of-life communication skills, listening to PowerPoint talks, role-playing the breaking of bad news, speaking to "simulated patients" — actors with scripted responses to my cancer diagnosis. And I've left each course profoundly disappointed.

It's not to say they are bad; they just don't seem to be designed for the ICU. They use mnemonics and catchphrases that sound contrived, corny, and out of touch. The most popular of these, SPIKES: Setting up the interview; assessing the patient's Perception of their condition; obtaining the patient's Invitation to give them information; providing Knowledge and information to the patient; responding to the patient's emotions with Empathy; and finally, Summarizing and deciding next steps. SPIKES was developed for sharing cancer diagnoses and includes getting an invitation from the patient to tell them bad news — a preposterous way to open a conversation with someone in the ICU, where families can't just choose to forego difficult conversations. Yet these programs have been thrown into every which medical environment, from emergency rooms to ICUS, with little adaptation or study.

Faults aside, many smart groups have worked hard to train doctors like me to communicate more clearly. Atul Gawande's Ariadne Labs, in Boston, the Center to Advance Palliative Care, based out of New York City, and the SPIKES creators have all done wonders for closing the gap between medical technocrats and the dying patient.

Yet here I am, certified in end-of-life communication techniques, and still deeply unsettled by the death dilemma. I have downright nailed difficult conversations and still had families push away and deny reality. Eventually, frustration sets in and I drift away from my therapeutic alliance with death-denying families. I've felt I was abandoning them.

AFTER SPEAKING TO THE communications gurus, I was left with an unsettling question: If I was saying all the right things, in all the right ways, why wasn't it working?

I confided in Jessica Zitter, the paragon who is both a palliative care expert and intensive care doctor, that I hated SPIKES and rolled my eyes during communications workshops. Surprisingly, she was on my side.

"I've had plenty of situations where I have used all my skills and tons of time with families and the ending is still a disaster. You aren't going to win every single one. But you have to try to be patient, and try to get to that particular person and understand them. Maybe only three in ten people won't budge."

I brought up how resistant some families seemed; they just didn't want to understand the medical facts. But Zitter, like others, reminded me that it's not about facts. "If you sit down with families and have a conversation and really get to know them and create a relationship, that's what they want. They want to know their doctors care about them. Then the next day you can talk about goals of care and their beliefs and start to understand.

"Families are as varied and different as snowflakes. You can't make judgements about what they are saying without knowing them better. It's about the relationship. It's about getting to know them, then establishing goals of care."

It's also about the frequency of connection, Zitter said. Frequency shows them you care, that you're not judging them, and that you're there to support them.

"We don't have time to waste," she told me, "so we put [patients and their families] into a box, and there is a huge problem in doing that. You need to get to know why someone is making decisions you disagree with. Maybe it's not you, because you don't have time, but it can be a chaplain, it can be a social worker. Getting to know people at a very deep level before throwing up your hands is critical."

But sometimes, you do throw your hands up in the air. And Zitter isn't immune to frustration. "There are many days I'm stressed and busy that I also take short-cuts, where the mother says, 'I'm praying for a miracle,' and I say, screw it, I'll just intubate him, what can I do? But the more you do this work, the more you have difficult conversations, the more adept you become at them, and the more they go well. Once you see it, you can't really go back."

ASK ANY KID WHAT they want to be when they grow up and "palliative care physician" probably won't top the list. As for "pediatric palliative care physician" — yes, they exist — well, no kid has ever put that ahead of astronaut, police officer, or rock star.

But that's exactly what Nadia Tremonti does, day in and day out, in Detroit, Michigan. For the past twenty years, Tremonti has cared for children with complex health conditions, many of whom never survive to adulthood. Whether in clinic, hospital, or hospice, she humanizes the dying process, bringing meaning and comfort to parents who must watch their children bounce in and out of hospitals their whole lives.

I asked Tremonti how the death dilemma came to be and how we might dig our way out.

It was clear she had spent a lot of time thinking about it. "We've gotten to a state in society where it is bizarrely hard to know when someone is dead. . . . As a culture, people don't even recognize anymore what death is. Most people, when they have someone who dies, the person was either killed or the doctor screwed up. No one can acknowledge that they had a disease that was terminal."

To prepare families of chronically sick children for the end, Tremonti slowly builds bonds that she relies on when difficult decisions have to be made; it's how she can help a mother who has fought hard to keep her son alive for so many years to recognize the end before its unpleasant arrival and "flip the plan" from quantity of life to *quality* of life.

But ICU doctors like me don't have the benefit of long relationships with patients and families, strengthened over years of tough times, tested in difficult situations, and cemented in mutual respect. Building those bonds, Tremonti says, was traditionally the role of the family doctor, who decades ago would visit dying patients in hospital and liaise between hospital doctors and families, bringing important context and a position of trust to the table.

But that all began to change in the 1990s.

"Over the last twenty or thirty years, family doctors fell to the wayside. Reimbursement costs weren't rewarding for coming to the hospital, and the workload of their outpatient practice was very high. And electronic medical records don't all talk to each other; I work in three different health systems that each use a different record system. A lot of doctors were turned off by the EMR [electronic medical records], and a lot stopped doing hospital work. And the notes that you do see now, like discharge summaries, are so full of garbage, and you can't even find what you need to know in the forty pages. There is no true impression or plan, it's just a bunch of inaccuracies."

As hospitals digitized and became bureaucratic burdens, family doctors stayed away, distracted by the computerization of their clinics. Having lost the involvement of their family doctor, hospitalized patients and their families had to navigate the complexities of critical care on their own, finding their own voice and building relationships with doctors from scratch.

Tremonti explained the importance of her presence in the hospital. "Whenever my patients are admitted to hospital, I'll go around and often just do a social visit. I'm not usually making a lot of decisions, but I may just pop by and talk to the doctors about the patient's baseline or what the family thinks or what end-of-life conversations I've already had. On Friday of last week, I had three different patients in the hospital, one who is actively dying. I wasn't necessarily planning to have conversations that day, but I noticed that in the last two months one patient was in hospital three times, and it seems to me like there is a pattern here, and its time to ask are the good days outweighing the bad days. But if I wasn't there, those conversations wouldn't happen."

Tremonti observes how hospital teams focus in on each organ but lose sight of the big picture. "It is hard, especially in the ICU, where every specialist is looking at a different part and not necessarily the whole condition. Traditionally it was the primary care doctor who did that."

Tremonti tries to help ICU teams and medical specialists "telescope out" for a wider view. She recalled one girl with breathing problems. She went to visit the pulmonologist, who could only offer a tracheostomy and ventilator. The family didn't want that, but the pulmonologist didn't want to send her home, because she looked so unwell.

"So this is where we aren't doing everything. We aren't doing nothing, but we are stuck in the middle. We struggle a lot with defining dying and interpreting if the person in front of me is dying and should we allow that, or is there something they are struggling with that we can recover. A lot of people are uncomfortable defining the grey zones and deciding when to flip this."

Flipping the plan is a term I had heard a few times. Emergency doctors use it to describe the conversations they have with families of patients who aren't suitable for full resuscitation efforts. I've flipped the plan myself as a paramedic, when a young man with esophageal cancer who weighed about forty kilograms (eighty-eight pounds) was taking his last breaths in his bed at home. His mother, who was understandably beside herself, had called 911 because her son was struggling to breathe. Rather than rush him to hospital, I stayed in the house and administered morphine to relieve his respiratory distress. He died moments later, peacefully, at home, rather than in the back of a bouncing ambulance racing towards a hospital. It was, I think, one of my best moments as a paramedic.

But it's not always so easy to flip the plan from "resuscitate" to "palliate."

Tremonti described the frustration that can arise from our own medical successes. "A lot of these chronic diseases, we get [patients] to bounce back, maybe not to where they were, but the next time they come in, and you're like, 'Well, this time they might die,' the family [says], 'but you fixed them last time.'"

The point at which we should be flipping the plan gets more and more blurred. "You can run around in circles," Tremonti said, but at some point you have to "turn off the curative tap and turn on the palliative tap."

Very few families choose the natural-death path in pediatrics. In their hope that things will get better, most of them will have a feeding tube put in and a tracheostomy. "I don't think it's a wise decision, but most people do. And here we have a family who has chosen a palliative path that doctors often think is the logical thing to do, but it's not so easy. Sometimes people die too slowly.

"People have so little exposure to natural dying. It's common to have sudden death but not really slow deaths. With heart failure, they get a pacemaker, and then they get an LVAD [left ventricular assist device], so they were dying the whole time, but it's so medicalized that when those technologies fail, death then comes quickly. It's not that you're here one minute and then you're gone."

I asked Tremonti if she has tricks for communicating the *slow death*.

"I tell them what's going to happen. I focus on how the body shuts down. There is a process, but it can take days or weeks. I tell the family what normal dying looks like, gasping respirations, turning blue. They stop eating and then they stop drinking and then they go to sleep and then they die."

I asked her if she agreed with Brian Carpenter that doctors like me should adopt the tricks the oncologists use.

"In oncology, the diagnosis point is really clear, the staging is clear, the way they plan their imaging and chemo treatments is very clear, and you know if it's working. There are stop points, like this is the last chemo and there is no further cancer treatment." So the oncologists have an easier time, maybe, than ICU doctors, who are trying to sort out what technology might make you better and what might just make you die slower."

In the ICU, she said, I should talk about what I'm seeing, not what I'm doing, then sit down with families and explore with them what their priorities are and make note of that, because that's where my focus should be.

Tremonti also asks her patients about religion — "Are you someone who thinks more scientifically, or do you think of things in a more spiritual way?" — and then explores that with people. "Then you ask people, given what you know, 'What are you hoping to achieve, and what are you afraid of and wanting to avoid?' And whatever they say, these are openings. And that can be a helpful approach."

This seemed more up my alley than the scripts I had

been given in the past that seemed contrived and out of touch. I asked Tremonti to keep going.

"There are a lot of misconceptions out there. People think medicine can do things that it just can't. When their goals of care are that they won't die, that they'll get healthy, you have to negotiate those goals to be more realistic. If you can understand what motivates people, that's what their values are, and then you can use those values to come up with a more realistic logical plan.

"When you're meeting resistance, or families are making what seem to be illogical decisions, then you have to lean in and say, 'Okay, what are you using to make your decisions? 'Cause I'm not getting it.'

"When doctors think families aren't making the decision we want them to, we keep flooding them with more and more data and science, and in fact that has nothing to do with their decisions. My experience with families is that 99 percent of them make decisions based in the spiritual realm. Maybe the family is waiting for a sign from God. So you can ask them, 'What does that look like?' Maybe they give you some guidance: 'If his heart stops, then that's God saying it's enough.' 'Hey, that's what we think too! So when his heart stops, that's the sign you were looking for and we're going to stop.' You just got a DNR."

After speaking with Carpenter and Tremonti, I was a little less skeptical that communication skills could reduce acrimony in the ICU. I was becoming convinced, however, that it wasn't so much how we asked the questions but more a matter of asking the right ones.

It reminded me of cases in the neurocritical care unit at Stanford, where people with severe brain damage from strokes and trauma would arrive. Many of these patients had healthy bodies but damaged brains, and goals of care conversations wouldn't focus on survival, because survival was likely. Rather, they would focus on determining what an acceptable quality of life would be. Families would say, "She would never want to live in a nursing home" or "He valued his intelligence and independence" and, despite uncertainly around death, we could say with great confidence, "Oh, we won't be able to get them to a point where they can be independent." And for most families, that made the next step crystal clear. We would focus on comfort.

Still, to boil the death dilemma down to a matter of language seemed too easy. Doctors still needed to be willing to deploy the conversation skills being taught to them, and families still needed to accept that at some point the plan might need to be flipped, that palliative care was the only humane path forward. Language won't fix the awkward positions we find ourselves in, with both sides firmly camped on the edges of reality, hoping every patient will just get better, if only we try one more thing.

The death dilemma is about more than equipping doctors to better explain that the end is near. The doctors whose default response to a dying patient is to apply more health care must buy in to the notion that not every life can be saved, and our extreme measures might not always be as virtuous as we hope. In

aggressively advocating for more health care, we paradoxically place some people in a state of less health.

The dying journey used to be chaperoned by spiritual experts—priests and rabbis and imams. Now, it's
guided by overstretched social workers, a rotating cast
of bedside nurses, and physicians who can't seem to
comprehend why families don't understand our medical mumbo-jumbo. And while religious authorities can
be quite accepting of death, too many physicians are
instinctively programmed to repel it, bringing ambiguity to end-of-life conversations.

This is a complex bio-psycho-social problem that
isn't amenable to a simple solution, so I found it a bit
confusing that the experts I had spoken to seemed to
imply that if we could only train doctors to be master
communicators, the death dilemma would go away.
Catchphrases and mnemonics and workshops merely
scratch the surface.

But something deeper had emerged from my conversations with palliative experts, anthropologists,
patients, and my colleagues. Whether communicating
a prognosis or exploring hopes with a patient and family
for the remainder of the patient's time on earth, it still
felt like we were skirting around the crux of the matter.
The circumlocution left everyone—patients, families,
health care workers—still on the rollercoaster ride,
paradoxically talking about implementing palliative
care while celebrating micro-improvements and considering a menu of escalating technologies. For both
sides of the death dilemma, it was time to address the

elephant in the room and dig deep into our fears of reaching the end.

Even when a patient is riddled with ulcers that we know will never heal, we march on, afraid to admit our failures as doctors and face a family already devastated by critical illness. Wound ulcers occur in areas where gravity pulls bony parts into skin, decreasing blood flow and causing skin cells to die. Eventually the ulcers erode through the skin completely, then fat tissue, then muscles, and then bone. Looking into a late-stage ulcer, you'd think a mini landmine exploded, creating a deep crater.

But we keep going. More machines, more devices. More hope, more prayers. More suffering.

It's the only thing we know how to do.

Slow Codes End Quickly

DESPITE BEING PROGRAMMED ALWAYS to resuscitate, doctors and nurses have an innate sense of when someone is too far gone. In those circumstances, moral distress boils up, eating away at us. We view ourselves as complicit in the evils of a slow death — the pain, suffering, and angst some patients experience as they die slowly on machines that can't save them.

A code blue, usually associated with acts of medical heroism, is, when applied to the dying patient in the ICU, perhaps the most gut-wrenching betrayal of the Hippocratic oath to do no harm. The pain of chest compressions, the distress of a chaotic scene of yelling orders, the frenzy of needles and tubes being shoved in your body as you fade away, is just one step too far for many of us to handle. ICU teams have come to find workarounds to ethically fraught situations where doing "everything" to a patient who fears death would do absolutely no good and would most certainly deliver harm.

One of these workarounds is the "slow code." The slow code refers to a situation where a patient is coding—losing their vital signs—and requires, through their own expressed wishes or the demands of the family, that "everything" be done. Depending on where you work (or, in some cases, who you work with) this could mean different things. As a paramedic, there was no such thing as a slow code; every code got an enthusiastic response, ribs cracking as we pounded on your chest to beat your heart back into action. This was because we didn't have any time to assess the viability of such actions; we would arrive, jump out of our truck, and get to work.

But in the hospital, where the code could be predicted, anticipated, and fretted over, it meant the nurse might not call for help right away. The code blue team might not run quite so fast. The chest compressions might not be quite deep enough to eject blood out of the ventricles.

In the last ten years, the rules have changed. In many places, doctors are allowed to decide not to do chest compressions even if the family demands it, so long as there is a reasonable professional judgement that CPR will offer no benefit. I found it puzzling that when I arrived at Stanford, different attendings told me different things about whether or not CPR was mandatory in full-code patients — some thought it was, and others thought it wasn't. Rules aside, withholding CPR is contentious, and to avoid the grief that can come with having to justify not performing it, many physicians will just run a slow code. Instead, so we can document that "everything" was done, we perform a half-assed CPR. This isn't necessarily less traumatic for the patient; perhaps it's just how us medical folk protect ourselves from moral injury.

But old habits die hard. I recently resuscitated a still-born birth, automatically cutting the cord and moving the flat baby to a warmer so my team could execute a "neonatal resuscitation" in a choreographed display of teamwork. Drilling a needle into the baby's tibia, placing a plastic tube down into his trachea, compressing his tiny chest. The baby, of course, didn't survive; he was never going to. But the emergency department is designed to act against all odds. And I didn't sleep for two days, guilty of the chaos I conferred onto "BABY, MALE99."

I WONDERED TO WHAT extent the medical industry was merely acting in response to families' and patients' fear of death and health care teams' fear of failure. Was all of the technology with which we'd surrounded ourselves just a way for us doctors to delay inevitable conversations about our own limits and ensuring customer satisfaction?

I asked Art Slutsky, the influential innovator of mechanical ventilators, whether technology had done more harm than good. The devices, he said, were not the problem; the devices save lives. But they must be applied judiciously and wisely. They cannot be indiscriminately applied to everyone who, in the case of respiratory failure, will die without a ventilator; they must be applied to people in respiratory failure for whom a ventilator can not only stave off death but lead to a better quality of life.

I realized that perhaps I had it all wrong. My career had focused on preventing death, but that's not the same thing as saving lives.

When I teach medical students about emergency medicine, I start with a lecture on adenosine triphosphate, or ATP. Made by metabolizing oxygen and glucose, ATP is a tiny molecule that powers cells to regulate their chemical composition. Without it, cells explode, organs shut down, and bodies die.

I tell medical students that every treatment in the emergency department is designed to help cells maintain adequate ATP levels: intravenous infusions, defibrillators, antibiotics, suction catheters, the works. If we can't get oxygen and glucose into the cells, the game is over. We fail.

But passing on this viewpoint that life can be thought of as chemical reactions is even more harmful than specialists trying to save a body one organ at a time. Our passionate drive to save lives has led to technological innovations that can facilitate chemical reactions that keep organs alive. We have a drug or machine for every organ (except the liver, which is just too complicated to mimic, and the brain, of course). In emergency medicine and the ICU, we rack our minds over lab results and radiology scans, desperately looking for a way to apply the drugs and devices in our toolboxes to fix the problem. But we don't often pause to look at the patient and consider their personhood.

A fear of mine was becoming clear: the death dilemma was at least partly my fault, because I feared failure as much as my patients feared death. While I seemed to be more in control of the ICU rollercoaster than anyone else, I still didn't have the sole authority to cut the power.

So doctors and families are both to blame for the death dilemma. Technology is off the hook, an innocent and necessary bystander made to seem problematic by the unwise actors who yield it. Ego, hope, and entrenched belief cloud our judgements, leading to well-intentioned actions with disastrous consequences for the dying patient supported by machines but left in limbo by those empowered to end their suffering.

Being confounded by our desire to improve our future medical capabilities plays into the challenge, but along with our well-intentioned use of technology we must also be able to recognize when that technology has had its chance to save a life. Once you realize the horse is out the barn, you don't need to improve the barn door.

The solution, it seemed, wasn't to understand the meaning of life more deeply. The solution was to be found in our fear of death itself. As a doctor in it to save lives, I needed to build an argument that could override the human brain's amygdala. I needed to construct an argument that death was a good thing.

PART III

Accepting Death as a Part of Life

CHAPTER 7

A Good Death:
How to Prepare for the End

The Default Option

FIRST, LET'S REVIEW THE law around what happens
when you can't speak for yourself—after a major car
accident maybe, or a severe stroke. When that happens,
doctors like me rely on a legislated hierarchy of "substitutes" to make decisions for you concerning quantity
of life versus quality of life.

In Ontario, where I practise, at the top of the hierarchy of substitutes who can speak for you is your
spouse, followed by your parents or children, then
your siblings. From there, the list works its way down
a somewhat arbitrary ranking of relatives and ends at a
government-appointed public guardian. Yep, a government bureaucrat could decide whether or not to pull
the plug.

That means it's important that you make your wishes known before they need to be known. "I don't think anyone wants a civil servant, however well-meaning, making those types of end-of-life decisions," Mark Handelman, the Toronto lawyer who specializes in health care law, told me. But only 25 percent of people have taken steps to ensure their wishes are known, and only 7 percent have spoken to their doctor. "You don't have a consequence as long as you stay healthy," said Handelman, "and that's the problem; death is uncertain as to timing."

Handelman says everyone needs to speak to their families about their end-of-life wishes and assign substitute decision-makers — or health care proxies, as some jurisdictions call them — through legal tools such as a written power of attorney, advance directives, or a living will. "The worst possible scenario is if no one is prepared for it and if the person who is sick has not expressed any values or beliefs about how they would like to see their last days managed. It's incredibly stressful on families and unfair to everyone who is still conscious."

Many times each week, I see the grief and tension these considerations bring to the families of my patients. They tell me they believe in miracles, or that the decision to pull the plug interferes with the will of a higher being. They often can't grasp the facts of what is going on and go through agonies in their attempt to come to terms with the impending death.

It's heart-wrenching to watch, particularly when

I know that the decisions they are required to make might have been less difficult if they could recall discussions they'd had with the patient about end-of-life care or could turn to documented wishes that described what the patient wanted done.

But having those conversations are admittedly awkward. To help, websites like the Conversation Project walk you through the best way to bring up the end of your life with your parents, siblings, and friends. It provides videos, guides, and other resources to help people work through the challenges of discussing the subject with those who matter most to them. The project, which coined the phrase "It's always too soon, until it's too late," suggests everyone aged eighteen and above choose a substitute decision-maker.

Lock It In: Put It Down in Writing

I first met Siobán when I was sixteen years old. I was an aspiring paramedic, and she was the leader of a youth group for paramedic wannabes. Firm but fair, she came across as the type of person a teenager might not like but certainly respected. Siobán mentored me, inviting me to ride along on ambulance shifts while I was in high school. It was with her and her ambulance partner, Rosie, that I saw my first dead person, in the cramped basement of a small house in southeast Toronto. We achieved a return of pulse, and that was the moment I became hell-bent on becoming a paramedic. I have no idea if the woman survived, but as paramedics, survival was far too distant into the future for us to care about. If you got a patient to the hospital alive, you had done your job.

Over the years, Siobán and I became friends. We would have frequent dinners and coffees in the Beaches district of Toronto, and I met her wife, Linda, and their cats. We found a steak house that became our favourite dinner spot, and there Siobán and I would tell war stories from our respective views of emergency care while Linda tried her best to follow the medical jargon.

Siobán and I both knew when to call resuscitations in the field, but we had no idea of the complexity of the death dilemma occurring inside hospitals, often with the very patients we thought we had saved in the field. That is, until Linda was diagnosed with a rapidly progressive early onset dementia.

Siobán retired early and cared for Linda around the clock while also caring for her widowed father at a veteran's home for the aged. In a matter of months, Linda needed to go into a nursing home, and a few months after that she was dead. I was startled at how quickly Linda had gone from being gregarious, kind, and full of life to being entirely debilitated.

A few months after Linda's death, Siobán and I met for breakfast at a diner in the west end. We talked about the end of life, how Linda hadn't been eligible for euthanasia because she was too demented to consent to it, and how painful it was to watch her, in Siobán's words, linger after her soul had seemingly left her body.

Siobán recalled the day she thought Linda's

personhood ended. "It was a Saturday when I visited with my friend Patty from New York," she said. "[Linda] had been bedbound for quite some time. She opened her eyes and took a huge gasp, looked quite shocked, and at that point her gaze became vacant and remained that way until she passed eight days later. At that point, I knew Linda was gone."

I asked Siobán what happened next.

"Now, we're just waiting for the body, for the corporeal matter to die. Whatever was Linda, her soul, her spirit, her energy, what made her human, that transcended to heaven. And then eight more days waiting for the body to follow."

Siobán wished she could have had the option to discuss euthanasia rather than watch the love of her life linger in a nursing home bed for eight days. "Once the brain is done, there is nothing left to save. So why can't the person decide ahead of time that once that's done, don't be wasting resources on keeping something that biologically has to die when the soul and the spirit has already departed."

It made perfect sense to me, but I wondered how, as a doctor, I could possibly operationalize that request. I asked Siobán how I could be expected to know that the soul had departed and we were just waiting for the body to follow.

"Ask me. Ask the POA [the person with medical power of attorney]. They'll know."

Not wanting to face the same slow demise she watched her dad and wife suffer through, Siobán

handed me an envelope. In it was a power of attorney
for personal care, a document giving the holder the
legal authority to make health care decisions. Printed
inside was my name. With it was an advance directive,
a legal tool that varies between jurisdictions but the
gist of which is that it places limits on what health care
providers can and can't do to you in life-threatening
situations. If you want to opt out of invasive technologies or painful surgeries, this document replaces your
own voice when you aren't able to speak for yourself.
Do-not-resuscitate (DNR) orders are a form of advance
directive, and are usually more brief, often offering
check boxes to guide things like CPR and intubation.

Having been witness to Linda's decline and week-long
coma, Siobán wanted to put in place instructions in case
that ever happened to her. She wanted someone with
power of attorney to be able to say, "We're done here."

"You know me," she said. "You know medicine.
You would know what to do, and you would follow
through."

Over greasy eggs and even greasier strips of bacon,
we talked about how life, for Siobán, was centred
around interacting with others and having the ability
to contribute to society. It wasn't about the brain stem,
which could make you breathe for eternity. It was about
higher brain functions, where you could think and ana-
lyze and find joy.

"Making that determination is the role of the power
of attorney," Siobán said. "And that's why my brother
is *not* my power of attorney. That's why you are. You

know me, and you and I think alike, and you can make that decision."

Siobán confided that she worried her brother would rely on his faith to make a decision that he could live with, even if it was outside of the clear lines she had drawn. "He didn't want to let Dad go, but as his power of attorney, I knew it's what he wanted.

"I knew what was coming, but my brother, Sean, had no idea what to do. Processing that was hard for him. He wanted a feeding tube put in, he wanted antibiotics given, but there was no sense in prolonging his life. That was hard on him. Not doing more was hard. He was having trouble coming to grips with the fact that it was Dad's time to go. He really wanted Dad to live longer."

When Siobán's dad broke his hip, she knew he made up his mind he wanted to go. He had surgery to repair the hip, but he never woke up from the anesthetic. It would take two full weeks before he died. "We had to wait for him to take his last breath. We were just sitting there with him waiting for the respiratory centre [in the medulla] to finally pack it in."

"That damn brain stem," she said matter-of-factly, followed by a short cackle typical of paramedics discussing dark topics.

Observing hesitancy in Sean made Siobán realize she had to come up with a sure-fire plan to ensure her own death was timely. "I remember being in the field on cardiac arrests with cancer patients, and families would have a DNR in hand and say, 'We aren't ready,

you have to try, you have to resuscitate,' and you just
shake your head and say okay. But with Dad, I was his
power of attorney for health decisions, so fortunately
Sean couldn't interfere. It was my call. And that's when
I knew Sean shouldn't be my POA. I don't think family
members can be objective enough to make the call
you want them to make. They inject their own values
or opinions or influences. So Sean might prolong my
suffering while he deals with his denial of my ultimate
demise."

Siobán could not have been more right. Time and
time again, families in the ICU are able to clearly articu-
late that "Mom would never want this" yet can't bring
themselves to let go, to let those wishes be acted upon
by the medical team. It's heartbreaking to watch, and
morally distressing to know you're not in line with
someone's expressed wishes. Generally, though, ICU
doctors will capitulate and give families more time
to come to terms with reality. "It's not that we don't
love each other or respect each other, but there is a
detachment when you don't pick your family. There's
an objectivity and intellectual process that you can go
through that Sean can't."

So having a power of attorney is essential, but it's not
failsafe. If your POA changes their mind, you could find
your carefully considered wishes tossed aside. "I knew
you would do whatever it takes," said Siobán, "get me
on a plane to Amsterdam, whatever needed to be done
to help me die if I was in the same boat as Linda."

Siobán remembered patients from her time as a

paramedic who had do-not-resuscitate orders and a plan to die in their home, but the family called 911 anyway. "On the road, I'd try to work with the family when they said, 'No, no, I'm not ready for them to die.' I tried to negotiate, to set limits. Maybe we'd try a bit of CPR but not intubate. We'd have a conversation to try to stick to the original plan and honour that patient's wishes.

"Most people don't witness dying. You can have a plan to go home with your terminal cancer, have the documentation and the plans in place, but when the moment comes, families panic.

"I remember one of the last ones I did. I remember hearing from the kitchen that 'I'm not ready yet,' even though there was a DNR. The wife knew it was happening, but she wanted a little more time to get emotionally ready. How is that fair?"

I asked Siobán what she thought about so few people having a power of attorney and directives expressing their wishes at the end of life.

"People are slowly becoming more self-determined towards the end of their life. They don't want to see their estate dwindle to nothing, being shelled out to hospitals and nursing homes, just to linger around. That money could be put to much better use for other charitable activities rather than keeping me alive when there's no hope of recovery."

Going Analogue: Palliative Care as an Alternative to Digital Machines

I'm usually late, but for some reason I was early on the first day of medical school. I took a seat towards the back of the large lecture hall. The room slowly filled with students the way magnetic balls fill a space: the distance they maintained between them slowly shrinking as the ratio of students to seats became smaller.

A guy sat down next to me and introduced himself. Chris Blake was a preppy kid nearly a decade younger than me. He had just returned from Oxford, where he'd lived on canned beans while completing his master's degree on laughter, an area that somehow qualified him to the title of anthropologist.

Chris and I would become good friends and eventually roommates. We were fairly different: I was a loud, to-the-point, no bullshit guy who just wanted to get through the day so I could go play on the helicopter overnight; Chris was a diplomatic fence-sitter who seemed incapable of being offended, which was easy because he hardly seemed to have a position on anything.

We were an odd duo, but we got along really well. He helped me mellow out, and I helped him grow a pair. Our house was known as a biohazard zone, neither of us very inclined to do dishes, vacuum, or dust the baseboards, which my mother told us we should really be doing every once and a while.

So it was no surprise that Chris and I would end

up on opposite sides of the medical world. He did a fellowship in palliative care at Canada's premier cancer hospital, and I did my ICU fellowship at America's Most Expensive (not really) Hospital.

Yet we often compare notes, because our jobs are in fact awfully similar. We'd both selected a career in which a vast number of our patients die under our care. But Chris doesn't see the death dilemma the same way I do. When people receive a palliative care consult, it's usually because they have a grave diagnosis and are looking for peaceful solutions to their symptoms. Chris is rarely called to an ICU; his patients typically have advance directives that expressly decline ICU-level care.

"I don't run into the death dilemma in my work, because in what I do, we kind of provide patients with guidance and the opportunity to plan in advance so that they don't end up being in this uncertain limbo between life and death," he told me.

The historical model of palliative care, Chris explained, was that oncologists and surgeons would do everything possible until there was nothing more to do, at which point palliative care would be called to come in and hold someone's hand and give them morphine. But the new model is different. Now, palliative care teams meet patients much earlier in the illness trajectory and provide them with a coach or person who can guide them through their journey and explore their values, what brings joy to their life and what things they wouldn't find acceptable. "You try to explore with them what medicine can reasonably accomplish and to what degree their goals are aligned with what's possible, and that's a long-standing conversation that evolves," he said.

Some palliative care patients will go on to be cured and discharged from Chris's care, while others will die, and he'll follow those patients and care for them right up to the end.

"I have my own personal biases about what might be good or bad for people, and I think that's based on my experiences as a physician and also as a family member of people who have received care and what my personal preferences would be," he said, "but I try to come in without an agenda. But what's achievable is dependent on what that individual's values are."

I asked him how he responds when patients say they want "everything" done.

"You have to explore why. Why do they want that? Maybe they haven't been that present in their family member's life, and they haven't seen the slow deterioration and suffering Mom has gone through, but they arrive and say keep them alive because they are feeling a sense of guilt or regret about not being there. Whereas the family member who has been around says, 'No, this has been enough suffering, let them go.' Or maybe they have a religious belief and say, 'We need to give every moment possible for God to work his miracle, for his intervention, so that this person can live again.'

"Come in to these conversations with a really curious mind and try to really understand from family members what they are hoping for from tech interventions. Only then can you really address their concerns."

Chris gave some examples of what people tell him when he digs deep. Some people want to live to a certain date, like a granddaughter's birthday, and are willing to go through a lot to get there. But if the reality of their condition won't allow that—say if they've got metastatic breast cancer with a bowel obstruction that isn't surgically treatable—there is a point where he has to tell them that if they continue to push themselves too hard they'll find themselves in the ICU.

"Some people, they accept that level of care, but most people don't." The vast majority of Chris's patients know they are dying and don't want to prolong the process. They value relief from nausea, reduction of pain, and easy breathing. They ask for medications that keep them clear of mind and free from anxiety so they can enjoy company.

I asked Chris how he manages to guide so many of his patients away from the ICU.

"Honestly, my advice is that you have to spend time with them. Time is a commodity. In the ICU there's not a lot of it, but it's our greatest tool. I was on call one weekend and came to see a patient who was actively dying, and her oxygen levels were so low the team wanted to intubate her. She was a full code. I spoke to her son for an hour, and we talked about the story of his mom's life and what was important to her. She was a woman of the church and always believed God would intervene to allow her to live longer, so no one had made her a DNR. I asked her son if she would still want to wait for God's intervention knowing that the doctors had nothing left to offer.

"He said, 'No, she would never have wanted to be on a ventilator, she would never want that.' So I flipped her from full code to DNR, and she died peacefully with her son at her side."

Sometimes, Chris says, all you have to do is give the family permission to let go. "I ask them about all the new information that's come to light, and if the patient had that information, do you think they might change the wishes they had expressed earlier when they were well. Most say that if the patient were part of the current conversation, they wouldn't want ICU, wouldn't want technology to prolong the inevitable."

This reminded me of one of my most useful phrases when people are on the ICU roller coaster: "Today is different from yesterday." Often, patients ebb and flow and their families see them worsen, improve, then worsen again. Families often say to me, "Last time, they bounced back." It can be humbling to see people perk up when I thought they were goners. But then, the ICU roller coaster keeps going, and eventually I find myself out of options and saying to hopeful families, "Today is different."

Chris drew out a graph he uses with his patients. On the x-axis was "time" and the y-axis was "quality." Everyone wants more area under the curve, both quality and quantity of life. But it's not just about how long they will live. At some point, the line may fall into negative numbers on the y-axis.

"I am a big believer that there is a negative quality of life."

Chris and I spoke about the horrible "negative quality of life" we have both seen in the ICU. He told me about a visit he had to a water treatment plant in high school. "The water guy said that he worked at the end of the line. If a dentist set up shop and dumped chemicals down the sink, he would know about it and they could work their way backwards and pinpoint the drain. The ICU is like that," Chris said. "You're the water treatment plant. Everything that goes wrong in the health care system, at some point it gets to you. You can work your way backwards and try to fix it. If you have time."

I asked Chris to work backwards from the ICU and identify the root cause of the death dilemma.

"Society has lost touch with dying as a part of life, and we need to remind people that death is a thing that comes for everyone and we need to think about it and be prepared for it. In Kerala, India, they deputized volunteers across the state to be involved in caring for people towards the end of life, and they have had incredible outcomes in terms of making people aware of death and dying."

Chris was hopeful about the future. He said palliative care is still a young specialty, but also a hungry one that wants to make sure everyone who needs a good death receives one, and that through ongoing education and advocacy, the future looks bright: fewer people will want to be kept alive by machines because they will choose a palliative care option instead, and probably live longer and better for it.

"Our generation is seeing our parents go through these bad deaths, and I think they'll be more accepting for a palliative approach to end of life. I think we are going to move culture and society to a point where death is not as alien and strange as it has been. I can tell you that there are lots of patients who I speak to about resuscitation, and they say, 'Oh, God, I saw my dad go through that. I would never want that for myself.' But you have to reach them upstream. By the time they end up on a ventilator, you've missed the boat."

Chris was emphatic that you can't convince everyone to accept death. "I've had patients where it's clear they will never accept death, and as long as I feel they are educated about their options, I can't hold myself to the expectation that everyone will get the death I want for them. But most people are persuadable."

I told him I didn't feel I was very good at being persuasive. Too often, I felt I gave in to forceful families not ready to accept the reality facing their loved one lying in an ICU bed.

That was the difference between our jobs, said Chris. "I'm not trying to save their life," he told me. "I'm trying to make their life worth saving."

Flipping the Plan: How to Let Others Go

When people get sick quickly or unexpectedly, or when they get sick but haven't had time to process that they're dying, there often isn't time to discuss goals of care. These unexpected emergencies lead to 911 calls and emergency department visits, where resuscitation-focused paramedics, nurses, and doctors rapidly respond to slow heart rates, low oxygen levels, and failing organs.

I don't see how this can be avoided. Indeed, most of the time, it's quite right to throw everything you've got into saving someone who has unexpectedly and suddenly started to circle the drain. As a paramedic and a physician, I saved many lives with the rapid application of medical technology, shipping people off to the ICU with a pulse while high-fiving my team for a job well done.

But now that I'm in the ICU, I'm seeing the consequences of these "successful" resuscitations. Patients who don't wake up. Patients who need more drugs than my pumps can deliver into their fragile veins, or more air than the ventilator can blow into their sick lungs.

This is the part of ICU care that Randy Wax extolled when he encouraged me to get into the specialty; the blend of resuscitation and palliation. Like emergency doctors and paramedics, intensive care teams want to save lives. We often continue the aggressive, tech-heavy approach started downstairs, not sure which way things will go. But as time passes, the trajectory becomes clearer: patients will either improve or deteriorate further. When the latter happens, it's time to shift the mindset from resuscitation to palliation, to flip the plan.

I first heard the term "flip the plan" in Nova Scotia. Paramedics would respond to nursing homes to haul demented, frail centenarians to hospital after a fall or because they had a fever. This was, in a word, cruel. The pain and confusion caused by a bouncy ambulance ride to be poked and prodded in a loud and hectic ER was viewed by the paramedics as torture. (I can pretty much guarantee that if you are sent to an ER from a nursing home, you will get blood work and a CAT scan of your head.) The paramedics developed language to speak to families about the goals their loved ones might have, and often this resulted in flipping the plan: instead of being rushed to hospital, the patient would be made comfortable and cared for in their own bed.

In the ICU, the plan flips too. We start out in full resuscitation mode — in it to win it. At some point, if the patient is not getting better, and it's evident they're not going to get better, we give up, though we don't say as much. With nothing to add, and the numbers all going in the wrong direction, we dance around the matter with families. Understatement: "It's not going well." Foreshadowing: "She's not responding to our therapies." Contemplation: "I need you to start thinking about what he would want." Mic drop: "I'm sorry, but she's never going to wake up." As you've read, those conversations can be full of tension. Families disagree with doctors. Lawyers go to court. A judge makes a decision. Everyone appeals.

While infrequent, these breakdowns are incredibly damaging. Doctors like me must dissect these horrific degradations in the patient-doctor relationship and commit to better communicating the realities of technological and scientific limits. Incorporating evidence-informed strategies in our communications is not a panacea; families must meet us halfway and openly hear what we are saying, even if those words are hard to hear.

Don't get me wrong—often, these challenging conversations go well, and families understand that the end is close, weighing their own hope against the wishes of their dying loved one. When families decide that the plan should flip from resuscitate to palliate, my job changes too. It becomes my responsibility to ensure that patients in my care with no hope of recovery and burdened by critical illness don't suffer from pain or anxiety until the moment of their death.

How to Get Off the ICU Roller Coaster

You can get off the ICU roller coaster a couple of ways. First, you can go full throttle until your heart gives out despite all the drugs, shocks, and chest compressions in the world. Sooner or later the resuscitation team will decide they've had enough, look up at the clock on the wall, and shuffle away. Second, your brain can swell until blood can't get in, and you'll be pronounced brain dead (also known as dead), at which point someone will schedule a time to turn off whatever machines are supporting everything below your neck. Third, you can choose to assign people in your life, and arm them with documentation, to make sure you never end up on technology to begin with and instead have a doctor like Chris Blake provide symptom relief and comforting therapy until you pass away. And fourth, you (or more likely, someone acting on your behalf) can flip the plan, at which point we'll keep you comfortable (and probably comatose) while the machines are peeled off and you die naturally.

My friends and I have discussed tips on helping people in the ICU die comfortably. When you're in this line of work, it's the kind of chat you might have over lattes. One friend likes to inject lidocaine to numb the veins before administering a sedative called propofol, which alleviates anxiety. Awake patients say propofol "burns" as it enters the IV cannula, and since no one really knows what's going on inside a comatose patient's head, why not numb the vein first? Another suggests a squirt of glycopyrrolate, if the nurses can find it, to dry up saliva and prevent gurgles commonly called the death rattle, which families find distressing. All of us around the coffee table take this seriously; we want the transition from alive to dead to be a comfortable one, both for the patients and their families, who often sit and hold vigil in the final moments of their loved one's life.

Recently , I arrived in the ICU at 5 p.m. for a night shift. "Oh, thank God it's you," said the charge nurse, who told me a patient needed "withdrawal" once all family members had gathered (some were flying in to be there). Turns out I have a reputation for being really good at killing people, and if anyone cares more than I do about a peaceful passing, it's the nurses I work with.

Saying I kill people isn't exactly true; at least, it certainly isn't the right legal term for it. We use doctor speak — an ethical principle called the doctrine of double effect — to get the job done. I order doses of sedatives and narcotics to alleviate anxiety and pain, ease respiratory distress, and prevent gasping and choking. But those drugs also lower blood pressure and breathing rates, a combo that can often push critically ill patients past the line. Since I prescribe these medicines under the principle that the patient prioritizes comfort over prolonged life, the side effects are tolerable (some might say they are even desirable). Double effect means that, even if the drugs are likely to hasten their death, as long as the intent is to provide comfort, it's allowed.

Practically speaking, it's halfway between what Chris Blake does in his palliative care practice and what Ashley White, who you'll meet very soon, does as a euthanasia provider.

On one occasion, an experienced ICU nurse I've worked with took it one step further when she suggested turning a patient on their side to adjust a pillow or change the bed sheets, knowing that even subtle movements can push people over the line. "Why prolong their suffering?" she said in a tone that only experienced ICU nurses possess.

Once the decision to palliate a patient who is in terrible agony has been made, the art of medicine shoves science out of the way. Recently, we've had a strong new focus on the patient and family experience of dying in the ICU. What was once a set-it-and-forget-it order of strong drugs to essentially (but not technically) euthan-ize a patient is morphing into a social experience for patients and families once the plan is flipped.

In this way, people have a little more control over the way they die in the ICU, the way Chris's patients have control, or how those who chose euthanasia can pick the time and place and playlist for their death. The challenge is that ICUs are hectic at the best of times, and most of us don't have time to tend to death the way we would like.

But that's changing.

In an effort to attend to human suffering and culti-vate relationships among patients, family, and ICU staff, one end-of-life idea is to grant dying wishes.

The 3 Wishes Project is a creation of a team at St. Joseph's Healthcare Hamilton, led by ICU legend Dr. Deborah Cook, a veteran intensivist and scientist where I trained at McMaster University. Intended to make dying a little less miserable by creating meaning-ful memories of one's final days, the project has helped honour the dying and ease family grief by facilitating impromptu guitar sing-alongs, or visits by a patient's beloved dogs, or reconnection with lost relatives. For some, weddings have been moved to the hospital, while for others artsy keepsakes have been made.

I was able to catch Deborah on the phone while she was cooking dinner to ask about why the 3 Wishes Pro-ject was born.

"It was as recognition that something was missing from end-of-life care," she told me. She described a death-denying ethos still very much alive in many ICUs. "To have a natural death, an ethos that has been a part of humanity for ages, is not really a characteristic of modern day intensive care units, so I was motivated to help to bring back humanism to the table, because something was missing."

Researchers tracking the project have interviewed families and caregivers of 730 terminally ill patients about their experiences with the program. "These largely simple gestures, the kindness, the encouragement of these thoughtful activities at the bedside bring comfort to those left behind," Deborah said.

Over the past seven years, nearly all of the 3,400 wishes made, by more than 700 patients, have been granted. On average, wishes cost only five dollars apiece, and most cost absolutely nothing. None costs more than two hundred dollars.

Deborah has praise for the very technology that can make dying so difficult. "Technology has progressed in an exciting way, almost unabated, and created new possibilities for interventions that hopefully do more good than harm. In the exciting journey of modern medicine, there has been a parallel shadowing of the importance of holistic care, and humanity doesn't always have a place at the table when people are severely critically ill," she said slowly.

"The 3 Wishes Project is about the importance of humanism, the importance of caring for dying patients in the ICU, and remembering who they were before their critical illness, especially since it can be a stark technological setting," Deborah said. "In the end, it's often the simple things that matter most."

Euthanasia and Its Limits

Controlling whether doctors and nurses try to save your life or let you go is one thing; requesting that your life actively be ended is another. Euthanasia has become more popular since the Netherlands first legalized it in 2000. Since then, jurisdictions in nine countries have followed suit, including nine U.S. states and Washington, D.C.

Dr. Ashley White is a jack of all trades, one of Canada's many rural generalists, bouncing between small towns and cottage hospitals, delivering whatever care is needed to the rural population just south of Algonquin Park, Ontario, about three hours north of Toronto. She delivers babies, anesthetics, and euthanasia. She works in a family doctor's clinic, in a walk-in clinic, and in a Botox clinic. She does both primary care and emergency care.

Ashley and I went to medical school together. We were both in the geriatric club, meaning we were approaching thirty years old when we started. And we both had real-life experience before med school, me on the helicopters and she in health roles in Kandahar, Afghanistan, where she almost got blown up by a roadside bomb, and in Ottawa, where the frustrations of the federal public health bureaucracy were more than she could take. She fled to medical school, hoping, like me, that as a doctor she would possess more agency to help transform a broken system in need of brave and urgent fixes.

Being almost blown up in a war zone must change your perspective on time, because every injustice Ashley identified in medical school became an urgent crisis requiring action. She would quickly call out peers who lacked sensitivity or exuded privilege, chastising young medical students who had never worked a day in their lives and benefited from wealthy upbringings. This made her a bit of a pariah, but I loved how she wore her heart on her sleeve.

More importantly, Ashley was always right, if not gentle, with her observations. I admired her for hitting the nail on the head time and time again. While she and I almost always agreed, I was less committal, more diplomatic, and questionably about as effective as she was at making a point, but she seemed more earnest in her convictions. She became someone I deeply respected and with each passing day wished to emulate a little more.

We lost touch after medical school, as her life took off with a child and a rural practice that had her essentially on call twenty-four hours a day, seven days a week, but I called her up because she is now an expert on euthanasia, or, as Canadians call it, medical assistance in dying, or MAID. MAID has been legal in Canada since just after Ashley and I graduated, but just because it's legal doesn't mean MAID isn't controversial in Canada, and it's still not easily available.

204 · ACCEPTING DEATH AS A PART OF LIFE

When Ashley arrived in her hometown of Bancroft, Ontario, after her rural practice residency, she was one of only a handful of doctors for a population spread across hundreds of miles of rural roads. No one provided MAID services, so she taught herself how (she literally googled it). Having witnessed first-hand the utility of MAID, Ashley now drives hours to patients in want of a dignified death. She has taught herself the art of killing, an art she practices about once each week.

I asked her why MAID is necessary when we have palliative care doctors like Chris Blake, who can minimize your symptoms while your disease takes its natural toll on your body.

"Continuing to live can be a form of harm," she told me. "The process of dying is where you find dignity, not in the death itself. Relief from suffering is what's valuable, not the act of dying. The cases that are the most difficult for family members and patients are the ones where I have to say, 'I'm sorry, you're not eligible.' Those people say to me, 'Are you sure? Can you come back in a month?' They are so desperate to die. But it's not one or the other; I deliver MAID, but I also provide palliative care. You can have both. Often, good palliative care means people don't want MAID right away. But there comes a time when they are suffering too much, despite all that palliative care can offer."

Ashley told me the story of one man in his fifties with metastatic lung cancer. His cancer had spread to his brain and liver, and his oncologist had told him he had no treatment options. He was going to die. The man got in touch with Ashley to ask her to help him do so.

"He came to me, and I said, 'I'll make sure you have access to MAID and palliative care. You are eligible, and when you feel like you want to die, let me know, but you need to understand that you must be competent at the time.' It was very clear.

"And then I got a call a few months later, and one of the home care nurses said he was getting foggy. So I called him into the office, and he came in and he didn't know where he was, he didn't know who I was. He was gone. I looked at his wife and said, 'He's gone, isn't he?' and she said yes. So I had to tell them that I couldn't help him die. I gave him the best palliative care I could, but he continues to suffer and fall and seize and all sorts of awful things. He didn't want this, I didn't want this, but he's not eligible under the current legislation that prohibits advance directive for MAID.

"Why couldn't I just register his wish a few months earlier? Now he's miserable, he's dying, it's time for him to die, we're all in agreement with that, but I'm not allowed. So he suffers. I've seen this happen time and time again. When people come to me and ask to die, they have not taken the decision lightly. They are clear, and they have been for some time quite often."

I asked Ashley to tell me about the patients who seek euthanasia.

Usually, it's a terrible cancer diagnosis, she said, but sometimes it's a progressive neurological disease. Often they are older, with independent personalities and a fear of being dependent on others for things like toileting and feeding.

Some people have relapsing diseases, and at some point they are told that they've reached the end of the curative line and that it's over. Normally oncologists don't say that, but sometimes they do. So patients have often come to this conclusion on their own, because nurses and physicians are very reluctant to suggest it to people.

Ashley reviews patients' files before she meets them to discuss why they want her to help them die. "I know exactly what's going on, but I need to hear it in their own words.

"Inevitably, it blossoms into this really beautiful conversation about the purpose in their life, and this goes all the way back to their childhood, and I get this beautiful narrative of their whole life. This is usually enough to establish capacity, but sometimes we'll do formal evaluations. This conversation is normally reassuring to the family, and then we talk about the details.

"Where do you want to die, what music do you want to listen to, who do you want to be there. And then I give a spiel where I say, 'When I come to help you die, you can change your mind right up until I start to push the syringe, but once I start, it will result in certain death and there is no turning back. And then it will be lights out, and everyone will see you become very calm and restful. And then I'll inject another drug that will result in a very deep coma. And then your breathing will stop and your heart will stop.'

"On the day of, I don't spend a lot of time dilly-dally-ing. I walk in, and we have a little chat, and I say, 'Okay, would you like me to help you die now?' and without exception they say, 'Yes, I'm ready now.'"

I asked Ashley if anyone has ever backed out on her.

"Never. They are ready. They are dying, and they are ready to die. The reason I don't feel like a murderer is because these people are dying and they are ready to go."

Ashley was one of the first doctors in Canada to provide MAID and is a fierce advocate for it. She under-stands the data around who seeks assistance in dying and why about as well as I understand the data around ICU patients who linger while their families come to terms with the inevitable. I asked her about the differ-ence between Ashley's patients who ask for a peaceful death and my patients who ask for "everything." Her answer seemed obvious, but it blew my mind.

People who request MAID are more likely to be edu-cated, wealthy, and urban than those who don't, Ashley explained. "This population of people have more inter-personal resources. They have insight into their own experiences that privilege and choice afford. I feel that for people who have had agency in their lives, MAID is completely congruent with their experiences that they choose to die. Whereas the people who are banging on the drum of resuscitation until the bitter end, that's also a form of control, perhaps a form of control they have never had before. Poverty is the absence of choice, and if you look at this from a socioeconomic lens, the people who are torturing their loved ones in the ICU have a sense of institutional distrust for many good reasons. They think doctors just want to get rid of their loved ones. Others have worked very, very hard to get where they are . . . they have worked so hard that they want to keep fighting. And for religious people, who put their faith in God, [they] have never felt they control anything, so why would they control their own death? It's something they just leave up to a higher power."

So there is a strong link between the degree to which you lived your life with agency and your death philosophy.

I asked Ashley if she had any tips for ICU doctors to ease the death dilemma, based on her experience offering a peaceful death to dozens of people. Her approach, she said, is to have discussions with families over coffee or tea. "You need to hear their story. It establishes that person's humanity, and when the physician acknowledges the depths of this person's life and says, 'I see your family member as a person,' then they will be operating from a common understanding of what's at stake, and that's a person's humanity. Then, when you say, 'I see this person, I see what they stand for and what they mean to you, and yet I know it is over and I know that what we are doing to them is going to hurt them and it's not going to bring them back,' you'll have a lot of success."

Ashley and I spoke about the future of MAID, which is highly restricted in the few countries where it's legal. In addition to discussing the need for wider access (Ashley supports access to MAID as a human right), we talked about the severely restrictive legislation that constrains doctors like Ashley. The most critical failure of MAID, we agreed, is the restriction that you must be alert and oriented and competent at the time of MAID.

Too many people rush it as a result, Ashley said. "They say, 'I would rather not linger. I would rather give up good time, because I am so afraid of missing the window and lingering.'"

I was horrified, but it made sense. I asked Ashley how often this happens.

"All the time. All. The. Time. People should be able to assert the position that they would like their life to be ended in the event they become unable to make decisions. There needs to be an ecosystem where people can safely navigate MAID as an advance directive. This would be most meaningful when it comes to dementia. So many people say to me, 'If my body is good but my mind is gone, just let me go.' We have long-term care facilities filled with people who don't want to be here anymore. I know that because their loved ones tell me their hearts break to watch people sit in a chair and drool on themselves all day."

Our conversation turned to organ donation, which more and more MAID patients are requesting.

"Tissue and organ donation is really an urban thing," Ashley said. "It's elitist. If you don't live near the city, you don't have access to surgeons and operating rooms. There's a huge urban-rural divide. It's a privilege to have a death at home and be able to satisfy donation criteria.

We call the organ network with every case, but we're too far away. Most of my patients want to donate their organs, but to make that happen, they have to be admitted to a hospital two hours away, so they decide not to. They want to contribute to the greater good, but it's more important to them to die in their home. But if you could make it convenient? They'd be like, 'Sure, man, take my organs. Just make sure I don't feel anything.'"

I asked Ashley about the fate of people who are dying but can't benefit from euthanasia because of the restrictions of legislation.

"I had one man email me and saying he was going to walk into the lake and drown himself. So I had to call 911, because of my duty to report. The end result would obviously be the same as euthanasia, but the experience is night and day. The distress that a person would have to go through in order to die by suicide is extreme. Also, the dissonance between the survivors is different. Family members who witness MAID say it was far more comfortable and safer than they thought it was going to be. Whereas I know when I've received a call about suicide, which I've experienced twice as a child and twice as an adult, is that suicide is traumatic because it's not cognitively congruent. They could have done X, Y, or Z. It is so traumatic to everyone."

One day, Ashley thinks, the law will change. Requirements will loosen and allow people to have advance directives so they can have euthanasia later, once they lose their faculties, or whatever exactly their value framework deems unlivable. But until that time comes, she'll continue to work within the law to bring euthanasia services to all who want to take ultimate control over their own end. Maybe one day, euthanasia will be a part of my toolbox in the ICU.

FOR MANY, EUTHANASIA IS a way to avoid the pains doctors today can extoll on people as they near the end of their lives. Afraid to wither away, they instead choose a controlled — if not early — death, away from the institutions and machines that define modern medicine.

If only we could find a middle ground, the way Chris Blake and his palliative care colleagues do, without the divisiveness of having to declare your code status and pick which side of the treatment fence you want to reside on, or if only we could allow decision-makers, like Siobán, to make loving decisions for those they love that reflect the patient's values.

CHAPTER 8

Life after Death:
The Legacy of Organ Donation

A Legacy of Life

ONE OF MY FIRST interviews as a journalist was with a
retired teacher named Heather Talbot. Heather had lived
through every parent's worst nightmare. I will never
forget sitting in her kitchen, drinking tea with her, as
she told me with vivid clarity of the day her son died.

Early on a Sunday morning, she had been woken up
by her doorbell. "I looked out the window and thought,
'Oh my God, a police car.'" An officer stood on her porch
and said her son Jonathan had been in a car crash just a
few miles from their home.

Heather jumped into the cruiser and was rushed
to the local trauma centre, where she was met by ICU
doctor Damon Scales. "Jonathan had severe brain
trauma, and the doctor said he couldn't fix it," Heather

told me. "The next day, he said Jonathan was brain dead."

Heather didn't know if her son would want his organs donated. "It crossed my mind. I thought, 'Are they going to ask about donation?'"

But his sister knew; when the two had gone to get his driver's licence, he'd signed the organ donor card.

Heather began having conversations with her family, her rabbi, and an organ donation nurse at the hospital, and made the decision to make Jonathan an organ donor. He would go on to save four people's lives.

The organ donation nurse was a key player in Heather's decision. Most hospitals have a dedicated team of nurses who specialize in conversations around donation. In my hospital, these nurses are the only ones allowed to discuss the topic with families, because it's been shown that receiving specialized communications training—they go through hundreds of hours of simulated conversations and receive education on various religious and cultural views on donation—provides the best shot for having families arrive at the decision to donate.

I had worked with a few organ donation nurses in my ICU training, and I asked them to put me in touch with the province-wide organ donation agency, called the Trillium Gift of Life Network, to arrange a formal interview. A few days later, I ended up on the phone with Pam Nicholson.

Pam had been an organ donation nurse for ten years. She describes her job as helping families make a decision that the person in the bed would have made, and she is careful to point out that it's not her job to convince families to donate, just to help them understand the options and to guide them through a process of considering what the patient would have wanted.

"I'm also the voice of the people who are waiting. If we don't speak for them, no one else will," she says. In Ontario, where Pam works, there are 1,500 people on the organ wait-list, and every three days one of them dies because they didn't get their lifesaving transplant. In the U.S., a new name is added to the national wait-list every ten minutes, and seventeen people on the list die each day.

This tension—not wanting to pressure families while also aiming to facilitate as many donations as possible—is something donation nurses seem to tiptoe carefully around. The professionals who work in this area are exceptionally wary of damaging public trust by upsetting grieving families, so when I spoke to the Trillium organization's CEO and public affairs officer, I could sense some inherent discomfort as I tried to sort out the goals of the agency.

Pam was able to answer me more directly. "We want people to make the right decision with no regrets," she said.

Pam had statistics that showed families who chose donation didn't later regret the decision, and those who declined often wished they could go back and change their mind. She also had a ton of expertise in myth-busting: surprisingly, no major religion forbids a person from donating organs, though the justifications for allowing transplantation are in some cases rather creative.

The main reason people say no to organ donation, Pam says, is because they didn't know what their loved one wanted. But one in five registered organ donors have their wishes overturned by their loved ones, and this is often because they hadn't spoken to their families about their thoughts. This creates a bit of conflict between organ donation nurses like Pam, who want the patient's wishes honoured, and families who dig in their heels and allow good organs to go to waste.

In California, where I'm working now, the law forbids families from vetoing previously declared wishes to donate. Hospitals go ahead and take the organs anyway, something I found jarring at first. In one case, a family tried to get a court injunction against the surgeons, but the courts sided with the hospital. Back in Ontario, where I trained, similar legislation supports removing organs without family agreement in cases where the patient had registered their wishes to be a donor. But it's hardly ever used. If the family disagrees with the patient's wishes, which happens about 20 percent of the time, the organ donation agency, fearing erosion of public trust in the very idea of organ donation, prefers to let one body go in favour of staying out of the news.

This "family veto" dilemma vexes organ donation experts, who have yet to come to a consensus on how to address the challenge. Do we upset families to honour our patients' wishes, or limit distress and friction to maintain the peace?

Jonathan's mother, Heather, for her part, has no regrets. "Organ donation has given my life new purpose to honour him and keep his memory alive," she says of the four lives saved by her son's organs. I could see the relief she found in discussing the good that came from her son's tragic death. There was a spark in her eyes, a purpose that helped her push through the pain.

There was purpose in Pam's voice too when we chatted. She spoke eloquently and calmly, but also with a hint of desperation. I imagined what it must be like to go to work every day and talk to parents of brain-dead teenagers, desperately hoping precious organs can be kept alive long enough for the testing and allocation processes to run their course. I asked Pam if she had anything else that she wanted people to hear.

"Don't take your organs to heaven," she pleaded. "Heaven knows we need them here."

The Dead Donor Rule and Other Quirks of Donation

You might think, listening to Pam Nicholson, that agencies responsible for organ donation would bend over backwards to ensure their wait-list was as short as possible. But as it turns out, there are several rules that limit donation.

Organ donation agencies put public trust in the donation system above all else, and rightfully so. In the fifty years in which doctors have been taking human organs from one body and installing them in another, groups have acted to limit the science of transplantation. Just take the case of Dr. Wada, the Japanese surgeon charged with murder when he followed in Christiaan Barnard's footsteps.

One of the most unbending rules in organ donation is the dead donor rule, a seemingly straightforward policy that demands patients be declared dead before life-sustaining organs like hearts and lungs are removed. Intended to bring confidence to the public that doctors won't go harvesting organs from those who might live, the rule is nearly as old as transplantation itself.

But a closer look at the dead donor rule pokes holes in the idea that death must occur before donation can proceed. In many ways, practically speaking, the concept that a person must be dead to give up their heart is a doctrine that hinges unreliably on semantics.

To demonstrate the absurdity of the rule, people who are declared to be eligible donors but who haven't quite met the strict criteria for brain death must linger for an indefinite period off life support until their heart has stopped for five full minutes—an elapse of time that deprives the heart of oxygen long enough that sometimes it makes heart transplant impossible. Surgeons pluck out the remaining organs in the order of their vulnerability to hypoxia. Liver first, then lungs, then kidneys. It's a bizarre game that results in perfectly good organs being thrown in the trash. Some people's hearts stop as soon as life support is turned off; for others, it can take many hours. And despite my best judgement, I'm not very good at guessing just how long it will take. Two hours is considered the limit in Canada; if it takes longer than that to be declared dead after life support is withdrawn, all the organs may be deemed unsalvageable. A wasted legacy.

But the loss goes beyond the organs themselves. Families, often buoyed by the purpose donation offers in the face of tragedy, are devastated when organs meant to help others are deemed unusable. It's like the person died twice.

And in the case of euthanasia, battles have broken out over patient autonomy. Many patients who have decided to die in a controlled fashion want to ensure their organs have the best chance of helping others. But that would mean dying by organ explant—going into the operating theatre, being given general anesthetic, and then having the freshest possible organs removed— something that under current legislation is not allowed. About one percent of all hospitalized patients become organ donors, which is about the same percentage of deaths that occur by euthanasia in Canada. So if every patient who chose euthanasia were also able to donate their organs, we would double the number of organs available for that long list of patients dying of organ failure. As it is now, many patients can find themselves in a catch-22, forced to choose between the death they want and the death that will allow them to donate.

I called up Ian Ball, an ICU doctor and donation expert who argued against the dead donor rule in the *New England Journal of Medicine*. Vilified in certain newspaper reports for questioning the policy, Ian was a bit hesitant to chat on record with me, but when I told him what I was writing about, he accepted the opportunity to make his case.

In November 2017, Ian was at a national critical care professionals meeting in Toronto. Someone stood up during a breakfast session and asked, "Should we revisit the dead donor rule?"

"It was dead silence," Ian told me. "You could hear a pin drop. And the panel was quiet. People in the audience giggled, and he sat down, and that was that."

But one year later, at the same meeting, the dead donor rule came up again. "They asked for a show of hands—Should we revisit the rule?—and half the hands went up. So I think people are interested and willing to discuss this."

The whole concept of the rule is to protect donors from their physicians, who hypothetically may be more interested in the recipient than the donor they are charged to care for. But Ian questions the need for this level of protection. "Why would I place the needs of someone I have never met ahead of those of the patient in front of me? That's an extremely conservative perspective that ignores other conflicts of interest, like the reimbursement for each day you are in an ICU. It's just an artificial construct that makes people feel better, but it harms the organs. When you wait longer for people to die, the organs may be less suitable for donation."

This matched my experience working in several transplant ICUs. Often, when patients with new organs suffered complications, their surgeon would say something like, "Yeah, that doesn't surprise me. The organs weren't that good." In private, transplant surgeons have told me that organs from donors whose hearts have first had to stop aren't as good as ones that come from brain dead donors, who go to the operating room with a heartbeat pumping oxygenated blood to organs, keeping them perfused—alive—until the very end.

"I understand where they are coming from. They are very concerned with public perception." But, Ian suggests, it's paternalistic to make the assumption that the public accepts the dead donor rule in today's society. Indeed, when the public is surveyed about organ donation in general, they endorse actions that improve the health and availability of organs so long as there is transparency and attention to comfort.

"The dead donor rule is antiquated," Ian argued. "We need to trust the public as much as they need to trust us. People are more connected and more aware, and they want all the information." And for the record, I completely agree with him. If I were ever in the situation where I was going to die imminently, I'd want my heart snatched out of my warm, alive body so I had the best chance of it saving another life.

The legalization of euthanasia has brought some urgency to updating the dead donor rule. Canadian legislation says if you are receiving euthanasia, you must die by drug administration, which means you aren't allowed to have your organs plucked out while you're still alive. It's a pointless rule, many argue. You're going to die either way.

Ian told me about a patient who came to hospital to

have euthanasia and then donate their organs. It didn't go so well.

"Normally in euthanasia, we don't have an arterial catheter, so when a patient loses their pulse, they're dead. But the organ donation organization required an arterial line, and their blood pressure dropped to 22/10, but it stayed there for too long and the surgeons couldn't take the organs because we lost the window. But they were going to die; we had just administered a massive lethal dose of drugs. So to have to wait is just silly."

His hospital has since decided in similar cases to administer potassium chloride to paralyze the heart, avoiding the waiting game and heartbreak when people don't die quick enough. A few other hospitals do this too, but it's far from the rule. Ian told me, "We have tremendous pushback from pharmacists who say, 'You can't do that, it kills people,' and we're like, 'That's the point.' Patients want to die humanely and comfortably and in the best position to donate high-quality organs."

Nowhere in medical school did I learn that a blood pressure of 22/10 means you are alive; it's generally taught that people with a systolic blood pressure under 50 don't have palpable pulses. If you had this blood pressure after a resuscitation attempt in the field when I was a paramedic, I would have pronounced you dead, because you wouldn't have a carotid pulse, just like Ashley White would pronounce you dead if she was euthanizing you in your living room. But euthanasia in hospitals is treated differently, and both Ashley and Ian think that's unfair.

Other odd rules in the donation world are similarly hard to wrap your head around. One says that the ICU doctor isn't allowed to bring up organ donation until the patient or their family has agreed to withdraw life support. But many people aren't aware they are eligible for donation and would want to factor in the chance to help others when making a decision.

Ian gave an example. "The donation organizations are emphatic that you should never introduce the concept of donation until there has been a decision to withdraw life support. But in the time it takes to make that decision, someone may develop a pneumonia or complication that makes them ineligible, and then, when you bring up donation, the family says, 'Why didn't you tell us we could do that three days ago! We would have made a decision to withdraw more quickly so we could donate.' It's a tough situation."

This paternalistic approach is, of course, meant to protect patients. But it actually decreases their autonomy. The rule makes the veiled suggestion that people might choose to die just to help others but ignores how such an opportunity could be a legitimate and valid part of a person's complex decision-making process around the risks and benefits of continuing to be supported by technology.

Some people argue that it's okay to talk about donation if the patient brings it up first, but that lands us back in the area of privilege and differing levels of agency Ashley White, the euthanasia provider, spoke of; it's often the more affluent, educated, and supported patients who would think to ask the question.

In some extreme cases, doctors have gone to great lengths to get around the dead donor rule. Some patients are taken alive to the operating room to remove a single kidney or lobe of liver, permissible in alive patients because it doesn't cause their death, before being brought back to the ICU to have their life support discontinued. Others have provided anesthesia for euthanasia in the home, rendering the patient unconscious but allowing the heart to continue beating until arrival at a hospital later on.

New technologies are changing the way dead bodies are handled before reaching a surgeon to have organs retrieved. In a world first in early 2020, a Canadian effort led by Dr. Andrew Healey allowed a forty-eight-year-old man with Huntington's disease to be euthanized in his home while an ambulance waited outside. Once death was pronounced, a team rushed to place the man face-down on a stretcher and attach an apparatus to his mouth to insufflate his lungs, maintaining them as they drove the now-dead man to an operating room. Time from the man's death to when his organs were flushed with cold saline was sixty-two minutes, and within fifteen hours both lungs had been transplanted into a sixty-eight-year-old woman who had been dying of interstitial lung disease. Thirty-one days later, she was discharged home.

My friend happened to be one of the paramedics who transported the man to hospital. Despite the fact that he was transporting a dead body, it was, he told me, one of the highlights of his career. The chance to bring meaning to someone's death was inspiring and refreshing. But there were complications; legislation forbids dead bodies from being transported by ambulances, and it took some effort ahead of time to get all the approvals needed.

While the case is groundbreaking, it only works for the lungs; the other organs aren't salvageable after euthanasia at home. And the practice has been slow to spread; in the year that followed the first case in 2020, only two more cases in Canada came to fruition. (But in fairness, the COVID-19 pandemic emerged right after the first case.)

Another development in organ donation by people who have been pronounced dead in an emergency department involves attaching them to organ support machines until their families can be approached about donation options. Similar to the lung preservation technology used in the Canadian euthanasia case, the effort has led to remarkable results from patients I otherwise would have shipped to the morgue. Two-thirds of families consented to transplant, and 17 percent of those patients had lungs suitable for donation. All of the lung recipients were discharged from hospital alive. A key component to the effort is "ex vivo" technology, where the lung is attached to a life support system that allows it to breathe and receive perfusion. Blood gas measurements assess if the lung functions well, at which point the decision is made to either accept the organ for transplant or decline it as unsuitable.

THE MORE I DUG into advances in transplant technology, the more excited I got; so many lives can be saved through the gift of life, and our techniques to succeed at transplant are only strengthening.

Having thoroughly comforted me with his science-driven explanation of why dead people are actually dead, I wanted to reach out again to Sonny Dhanani, the pediatric ICU doctor and organ donation expert. On the phone, we turned our attention to the dying. I wanted to ask him about the dead donor rule. I told him I was struggling with it—that it seemed to be a matter of semantics—and that if I were dying, I'd want to get on with it and give my organs the best shot at saving someone else. He surprised me once more.

"I do not disagree with that. I do think that over time we will bend on the dead donor rule....Do I think I'm ready for that now? No. I think trust is still an interest, and trust in the dead donor rule is really important, not just public trust but medical trust too. I'm not scared of opening that conversation up, but let's not jump in with both feet.

"Keeping it in place is not that catastrophic. We have technologies and surgical techniques that are amazing. We have ex vivo techniques that resuscitate organs outside of the body until they can be transplanted. So the pressure to abandon the dead donor rule is less. On the other hand, as the public understands this more, they are demanding their autonomy in this decision-making process. They say, 'If I'm okay with this, who are you to say I can't donate my organs?' So if we can find a way to ensure that knowledge is there, it would be key. Also, the science is there. If we can show that there is no hope for recovery, and that when you die you die, maybe we can look past the five minutes. As soon as your pulse is lost because your blood pressure is too low, I can predict that you'll die with 100 percent certainty. So maybe the dead donor rule can become the almost dead donor rule."

The next ten years will be wild with technology, and within twenty years, Sonny thinks, we'll have an artificial heart or liver or kidney. "Eventually organ donation will become a moot point."

So much for legacy playing an enduring role in resolving the death dilemma.

I BEGAN TO THINK back to the stories I had heard about families being deprived of conversations about dying, either because the doctors were misguided by perverse "survival" metrics or because they emotionally weren't up to facing the situation. After speaking with Sonny, I began to envision myself at death's door; what would I want for my own organs, my own legacy? How could I blunt the pain of my family? How could I make something good come from my own end?

As I did research on organ donation and the gift of life, I came across other ways people can give from the grave, through donating their bodies to medical research, by being cadavers for a new generation of doctors, even by allowing forensic scientists to study how their body decomposes so that the science of decay can bring murderers to justice.

I began to convince myself that in the discussions at the end of life, conversations about what comes with death could be valuable; they could change the zero-sum game of adding technology to keep people alive, a game that assumes nothing good comes from the alternative.

As technology and society advance, so too does the opportunity for good to come from tragedy. As shifting death dynamics make more and more possible, paradigms of the past will ultimately be revised, allowing more people to find comfort in the legacy of organ donation. This will not only improve the dying experience of patients who are near death, but stave off the deaths of many more who can benefit from a better life by receiving organ transplantation.

I guess technology isn't that bad after all. Sometimes, it can bring meaning and purpose to dying, as well as the gift of life. In such situations, it really is a win-win.

CHAPTER 9

Do We Really Have to Die?

BEING A PARAMEDIC WAS an incredible privilege, but it was also remarkably frustrating. "Frequent fliers," patients who are transported with such frequency that every paramedic in a municipality knows the address by rote, would break my heart; complex psychosocial issues, like a lack of stable housing, unemployment, mental illness, and crushing debt, resulted in chronic health problems that I couldn't fix. On the helicopter, I saw more preventable injury than I could have imagined, again a failure, one could argue, of our society to build a safer world. The underlying societal failures that perpetuated misery on my patients were so infuriating to me that these frequent fliers were part of my motivation to go to medical school. Maybe with *doctor* in front of my name, I'd have more authority to advocate for lasting change. Sadly, my transition to the ER saw these same patients stuck in the revolving door of the emergency department—not sick enough to get admitted and too complex to help in a maddeningly chaotic and busy ER. When the opportunity arose to pause my residency to go to journalism school, I felt I had to pursue it; my toolkit needed more in it if I wanted to advocate for meaningful change.

On the first day of journalism school, my professor, Rob Steiner, told us all to ignore our expertise and "flip our assumptions upside down." Journalists, he said, were susceptible to making assumptions, and the only way to avoid the trap was to assume everything we thought was true was, in fact, wrong.

I thought this was insane. That is, until I committed to trying it as an exercise. My first story as a journalist came during the height of the opioid epidemic. Thousands of people were dying after overdosing on synthetic narcotics like fentanyl and carfentanil, which are far more potent than traditional narcotics like heroin and oxycodone. Coroners were being overwhelmed with bodies, and downtown hospitals were struggling to make enough space in ICUs for those who were resuscitated. The only upside, it seemed, was that brain dead overdose patients were young and often had healthy hearts, livers, kidneys, and lungs that could be transplanted into people with terminal diseases. Backlogs on organ wait-lists began to clear, and a few organizations even reported having a surplus of organs, some of which ended up in the trash.

Needless to say, this was a hot topic for the news media, and I was keen to be ahead of the curve. As a

paramedic and then a physician, I had long administered naloxone, which temporarily blocks the effects of
opioids, and marvelled at how just seconds after administering it into an overdose victim, they would start to
stir, to breathe, or wake up and talk. It was a miracle
drug, and many in the public health community viewed
it as we do fire extinguishers or defibrillators: something that should be available everywhere to be put to
use at a moment's notice by anyone around.

I wrote a pitch for a story about the need for government to get out of the way and update regulations and
policies so that naloxone could be more widely distrib-
uted. Rob read my pitch and asked, "Why is naloxone
so important?"

I told him about opioid receptors in the brain, the
pharmacokinetics of naloxone, cited statistic after statistic, gave anecdotes of places in Europe where this had
worked. He, as usual, was unmoved. "Blair, if naloxone
is so great, why are there so many deaths in places that
give it out like candy?"

Frustrated, I prepared to go back to my computer to
beef up the pitch and prove my point. But as I walked
away, Rob shouted, "Think like a journalist, not a
doctor. Flip it upside down and see what falls out."

I called the toxicologist at my university and began
our conversation with an apology. "Margaret, I'm so
sorry to bother you, but I need to ask: Public access to
naloxone would save thousands of lives, right?"

Of course it would, she told me. If this were a heroin
epidemic. But the newer synthetics being manufactured

overseas appeared too powerful for naloxone. In fact, she wondered if naloxone, which is highly effective in heroin overdoses, was a red herring, something we were pursuing as an answer when it might offer only a partial solution.

I was stunned. I started to dig into these new narcotics that were potentially resistant to naloxone. As it turns out, there was plenty to report.

The previous year, 2016, no one was celebrating the July 4 weekend at the Summit County, Ohio, morgue. Five apparent heroin overdose deaths in three days had investigators puzzled and overwhelmed. Autopsies were performed on the victims, but toxicologist Steve Perch couldn't detect any drugs in their urine or blood.

Perch inserted a powder residue found by police at one of the overdose scenes into his mass spectrometer and got a match for carfentanil, an opioid similar in structure to morphine but ten thousand times more potent and not included in most hospital or crime-lab screens. He had never heard of it, so he turned to Google.

Perch's discovery shed new light on the opioid crisis affecting America: criminal chemists were compounding opioids that were highly deadly — and undetectable — because their potency meant they could sell less physical compound for the same price as over-the-counter medications and well-known illegal drugs like heroin, making them more money.

Back then, carfentanil was known mostly to veterinarians — the drug is designed to sedate elephants and

other large animals — and after Perch secured a sample
of the drug from the Cleveland Zoo, about thirty-eight
miles north of his morgue, he developed a chemical test
to identify it in human body fluids. (He now networks
with toxicologists across the U.S. to survey for the latest
compounds, and when he and I spoke in 2018, he was
still struggling to keep abreast of a constantly changing
supply of deadly opioids.)

But when I was preparing to pitch a news story about
the need for wider use of naloxone, it turns out Canadian labs weren't even looking for the illicitly used,
naloxone-resistant carfentanil. And so I came to value
Rob's exercise of turning everything I believed in upside
down.

Which is why, in thinking about death and dying, I
decided to ask a bizarre question: With medical technology advancing so rapidly, do we even need to die?

Advances in Technology: Resuscitating the Dead

In Baltimore, and the world-famous University of Maryland Shock Trauma Center, victims of gunshots are not
treated in the traditional way I would treat them. The
moment they arrive, the bad cases get a cold slurry
pumped into their veins to replace their blood, and then
a ninety-minute timer is started. Cooled down, the body
needs little ATP, and thus little oxygen; it essentially
hibernates, like a bear in the winter. Without a pulse,
they are calmly wheeled to the operating room — no
yelling, no chest compressions, no ventilator. Trauma

surgeons then carefully repair what's been torn apart, and a heart-lung bypass machine is attached by the cardiac surgeons, who begin the slow process of warming and restoring blood volume.

What they've found by placing trauma patients in suspended animation is groundbreaking. There's little brain damage, little tissue damage, and a high rate of survivors.

Should this expensive, intensive treatment be extended to others? The pregnant woman with a large blood clot in her lungs? The child with a viral heart disease? The tennis-playing executive who suddenly collapses?

Well, depending on where you live, it may be.

In Paris, France, my friend Gérald Kierzek, an emergency doctor, does just that; rather than chill the body, he's put people onto heart-lung bypass (ECMO) machines on a subway platform, in shopping malls, and just about anywhere else. But he selects the patients carefully; a fair amount of intuition plays into each decision to go all out, and Paris is one of only a few places in the world routinely sending ECMO teams into the field.

In London, U.K., my friend Mike Christian, who was once an ICU doctor in Toronto, has saved dozens of lives performing a surgery in the streets that in the U.S. is only done in hospitals. He cuts open stabbing victims' chests on the side of the road where he finds them, searching for cardiac tamponade, highly pressurized blood constricting the heart so it can't beat anymore. Doing this in the field is something North American doctors have long frowned upon, but his patients are surviving. His record is three in one twenty-four-hour shift as an emergency response doctor.

Mike and I spoke about the death dilemma and how he decides whether patients with infinitesimal odds should be given a shot.

"We have to have humility about our ability to prognosticate. If we had a perfect way to say, 'Yes, this person will do well,' and, 'No, this person will not do well,' it would be easy up front. The more time I spend in medicine, the more I see that we are not that good at prognostication."

Mike worried that my solution to the death dilemma, to help families and doctors make choices to limit or withdraw life-sustaining technology, might mean a few would-be survivors could slip through the net.

"If we just stop resuscitating people," he told me, "if we make them DNR or euthanize them, then we have really good prognostic accuracy. We know they will not survive; it becomes a self-fulfilling prophecy."

Mike had stories that gave me reason to pause. "One of the things that changed my perspective when I came to London after being an ICU doctor for many years in Canada was there are patients that I've seen survive here, particularly head injury patients, who would not have survived back home, because we would have withdrawn on them. One guy in particular would give a lot of intensivists nightmares, and I've seen it with my own eyes."

Mike told me about a young man who came to

London to do a master's degree. "A few days after he arrived in the city, he got a major head injury in a hit and run. I intubated him in the street and he was comatose for months. Then literally one day he woke up and started responding. He's now home and wants to go do a Ph.D. in economics. I would have never thought that this guy would have ever recovered."

I agreed with Mike that it's not always clear who will live and who will die when we make decisions about implementing medical technology. I asked him how he manages to flip the plan when hope fades away after we've given technology a shot but it fails to work as we desired.

"I can't say that I'm fantastic at flipping the plan," he admitted. "But if you don't ever push the envelope with these patients, science is never going to advance. So how do you strike the balance between being very nihilistic and just saying we can't do it, we shouldn't bother, to saying we have to have these failures to help others down the road?"

We went back and forth on various thresholds, or decision points, that could be used in the ICU to decide to flip the plan, but we just dug ourselves into a deeper hole. Mike was emphatic about one thing, however: "Some patients are too young to die."

IT STILL ISN'T CLEAR to me where the line between nihilism and reality is.

What is clear is this: doctors around the globe are

pushing the limits of resuscitation, often with remarkable results. People who in Toronto would be declared dead, might in Paris or Baltimore or London go on to live full lives. The future of resuscitation is bright—but with ever-increasing efforts to pull people back from the brink of death, there will no doubt be more patients forced to face the consequences of too much technology, those for whom we tried to restore life but failed. For those who don't win the lottery and benefit from these extreme measures, they'll be stuck on the losing end of the death dilemma, having lost the technology gamble without outright dying.

This challenge is a big part of the death dilemma; in hopes of a good outcome, we press on, knowing that chances are slim. This has created a technology conundrum. As technology gets better, there is even more hope, more optimism, that resuscitation can save a life. But what happens when we roll the dice and lose?

The Technology Conundrum

The truth is, we don't always know with certainty if technology will turn someone around or prolong their suffering, and the two outcomes are not mutually exclusive. Some people may survive their life-threatening episode of heart failure or pneumonia, but after months or even years of rehab they remain deconditioned, unable to walk on their own or swallow food without the risk of choking. They may have a tracheostomy tube in their neck and require assistance of a ventilator, or have a feeding tube poking through their abdominal wall into their stomach to prevent aspiration, outcomes that are rarely discussed with patients when doctors seek consent to move forward with major surgeries or technologies that support life. Without a crystal ball, doctors focus on the short-term gains technology offers and the more definitive, predictable state of affairs should surgery or technology be declined.

It's not uncommon for a neurosurgeon to say, quite accurately, that a decompressive craniectomy — a surgery that removes a fifteen-centimetre-long piece of skull to allow a swelling brain to expand outward — will save someone's life. But equally true is that, for a clear group of patients, undergoing a decompressive craniectomy will not improve your chances of interacting with the world around you. It will stop you from imminently dying, but it won't lead to a better functional outcome.

Studies of critically ill patients often report patient outcomes using the Modified Rankin Scale (MRS). Many "life saving" interventions are very good at preventing patients from having an MRS score of 6 but do nothing to bring them back to 0, 1, 2, or 3. Some interventions do nothing but shift the outcome from 6 to 5, and I'd rather be a 6 than a 5 any day of the week.

0	No symptoms
1	No significant disability; able to carry out usual activities
2	Slight disability; unable to carry out all usual activities, but can look after own affairs without assistance
3	Moderate disability; able to walk without assistance but requires some help
4	Moderately severe disability; unable to walk without assistance
5	Severe disability; bedridden, incontinent, requires constant nursing care
6	Dead

At worst, they may be hospitalized for years or shipped off to a long-term care facility hundreds of miles away from their family. Daily visits become weekly, then monthly, and sometimes patients are entirely forgotten by the world they once knew.

Every ICU has its frequent fliers, its bounce-backs and chronic long-haulers, the patient who has been there for one hundred, two hundred, three hundred days. These chronic patients are often assigned a corner room, like a Gold member of a hotel, to have a nice view as they spend their life in the ICU. Enhanced TVs are often installed in their room, art and family photos hung on the walls, hospital sheets replaced with the comforts of the home linen closet. The nurses and doctors become friends with these patients while feeling a deep sense of pity for their miserable life confined to the wires and tubes that are ubiquitous to ICU residency. Birthdays are celebrated with songs and decorations. Eventually they reach the one-year mark, an ominous day that makes us wonder if we should get them a card or flowers or something else to mark the occasion.

All the while, the team wonders if any of the effort to keep them going is worth it; if only we had known, perhaps we wouldn't have tried so hard to save them from death.

I decided to call someone who was, I suppose, an authority on this conundrum; someone who was dead for three or four hours, only to be revived and, ultimately, be lucky enough to return to the way he was before he died. I wanted to know if he, had he had a say in this, would have rolled the dice?

In the early hours of January 15, 2016, twenty-one-year-old university student Tayyab Jafar, whose academic hopes were unravelling and who was suffering from depression, sent his friend a text message: "Sorry I couldn't be stronger. Love you. Goodbye."

Then, he took off his coat, washed down a bottle of pills with a can of beer, and lay down on a pier at the Lake Ontario waterfront in Kingston. The temperature was below freezing. Five hours later, he was found frozen to death.

Paramedics arrived quickly when they got the alert and were instantly mindful of a mantra drilled into us in training: you're not dead until you're warm and dead. They began CPR and rushed Jafar to Kingston General Hospital. There, doctors and nurses did over an hour of chest compressions and filled his body with heated saline fluid, trying desperately to raise his temperature, recorded at 20.8 degrees Celsius. But after an hour, his temperature had only risen to 22.8.

Kingston General is one of the few hospitals in Ontario able to put someone on cardiopulmonary bypass, a procedure equivalent to ECMO. But as in a lot of hospitals, the technology is reserved for those having open heart surgery. Many of them wouldn't ever entertain a phone call from the emergency department asking that a bypass machine be used solely to rewarm a dead patient, but it was Jafar's lucky day: a cardiac surgeon was both available and willing to give it a shot. With a nurse straddling him to pump on his chest, he was wheeled into the operating room, and Dr. Andrew Hamilton proceeded to place large plastic tubes into Jafar's arteries and veins so the machine could rewarm his blood at a rate of 9 degrees an hour.

About an hour later, Jafar's temperature was 28 degrees, and an electric shock was delivered to restart his heart.

"He was easy to get started," Andrew Hamilton told a local newspaper. "Nice young heart like that? Poof!"

Jafar's heart was beating. But the hypothermia was causing other problems: Jafar's blood wouldn't clot, and his lungs were filling with fluid. It would take over one hundred units of blood to stabilize him, so much blood it had to be shipped in from other parts of the province. The average person has about five litres of blood in their body; Jafar would receive ten times that volume in transfusions pooled from 134 donors.

Jafar would spend the next three weeks in the Kingston ICU before being transferred to his hometown of Oakville, where he spent another two months recovering in hospital. When I spoke to him, five years after his cardiac arrest, he had entirely recovered from his ordeal, with one exception: his right thumb couldn't give a thumbs up. Otherwise, he was back to full health. But his journey, he explained, had been long and painful.

"I was thrashing around. I had nightmares. The nerve damage was incredibly painful. With the trach, it sucks. Sometimes I'd forget how to breathe and panic. It was a weird experience."

I asked how it felt to have survived against such overwhelming odds.

He told me that after thirty minutes, most of the doctors wanted to quit, but there was one doctor in the emergency room who kept pushing the team to keep going, despite the odds. "It was just the one doctor who kept everyone going," he told me.

Jafar would be the only hypothermic cardiac arrest victim that Andrew Hamilton, the cardiac surgeon, had seen survive in his twenty-five years as a doctor. At most hospitals, they wouldn't even have the technology and expertise available to try. Without a crystal ball, Jafar's doctors went full steam ahead.

I asked Jafar, had he known what he would go through to recover, if he would have agreed to being resuscitated. The question seemed dumb even as I was asking it; how he regarded the months of painful rehabilitation depended to a great extent on how much the once-suicidal young man now looked forward to the life ahead of him, but his mental health had recovered.

"It was extremely challenging. All my nerves in my arms were completely destroyed. They said I might never have the use of my arms again. At the time, I probably would have said no.

"It's such a difficult thing to answer. In hindsight, I would have said yes, but in the moment, it's a different story. But you're not in the state of mind to make a rational choice, so it's not really up to you, it's up to the doctors. I can't really say how much doctors should throw at [people like me]. It's really up to their discretion. If you're dying, if the alternative is death, then they might as well do it. You just have to try, because if it doesn't work, [the patient is] going to die anyway."

I asked Jafar about people who are only half-saved, who don't die but don't recover the way he did either.

"It's a tough call," he said. "If you knew for sure that you weren't going to have a good life, I would definitely say in that case not going ahead is probably the better choice. But it's such a hard thing to know, because you don't know it's going to turn out. It's such a huge gamble."

A gamble. How many people end up with an MRS of 5, unaware of their surroundings and totally dependent on care in an LTACH facility, suffering alone and miserable for months or years before they die, so that one Jafar can return to school, hug his mother, and play video games with his friends? One in a hundred? Nine hundred and ninety-nine in a thousand? It's impossible to say. But I am convinced we are erring too far on the side of hope, celebrating the victories of the Jafars of the world and ignoring the tragic tales of survivors who live a life that is worse than death.

EVENTUALLY, THOSE STUCK IN the purgatory of the death dilemma will become dead-dead. If you spend a few months in an ICU, you'll end up suffering from complications: antibiotic-resistant infections, a blood clot in the lungs, bleeding in the brain due to the anti-coagulants used to prevent a blood clot in the lungs. The chronic ICU residents only linger for so long. About half of LTACH patients with a tracheostomy die within a year.

What about the rest of us? As we contemplate our own deaths, we can ask, Do we really need to die?

It's a question we've been asking since the dawn of time. In Greek mythology, Tithonus, lover of the goddess Eos, requested immortality from Zeus. Zeus granted this wish, but without the added gift of eternal youth. Tithonus would age and wither but never die; without any strength or mobility, he was locked in a room, where he babbled endlessly, lamenting his longevity and begging for death to take him.

The idea that technology entraps people, condemning them to eternal, miserable institutionalization, within reach of death but never crossing the finish line, haunts ICU doctors. I often wonder if I should attempt to resuscitate someone for fear I might get them to a point where they won't die but won't ever live outside the walls of a hospital. It's a choice that should really be made by them, not me, but too many times I've seen the unintended consequences of my heroic efforts. Am I being too pessimistic? Or is it egotistical of me to push the limits of medical science in the hope of outcomes like Jafar's?

I can't answer the technology conundrum; that job is entirely up to you. But if you leave it to the "system," you are playing the odds and spinning the roulette wheel. If the ball lands on black, you're dead. If it lands on red, you get a fate worse than death, like Tithonus, or the poor souls in my ICU who occupy the rooms with corner windows. That leaves the slots o and oo—the two green spaces on a roulette wheel—for a life like it was before, a life like Jafar's.

How Future Technology Could Disrupt Dying Even Further

It's hard to keep up with the pace of change in resuscitation. There will always be limits to what paramedics on the streets and doctors and nurses in the hospital can do to save someone's life, but some are looking further into the future, where I suppose anything is possible. They are asking not what might be possible in a hundred or a thousand years, but how to suspend life long enough to find out. Indeed, some researchers are asking if human existence needs to be tied to living cells at all.

Cryonics: The Tech Version of the Fountain of Youth?

In the 1990s flick *Austin Powers: International Man of Mystery*, Mike Myers's shagadelic spy hero is cryogenically frozen in the 1960s to await the return of his arch nemesis, Dr. Evil. When, thirty years later, Dr. Evil returns to wreak havoc on the world, Austin Powers is unfrozen. Shocked to be in a world where civility has replaced the womanizing times he relished pre-freeze, Powers gives us a glimpse of what it might be like if cryonics were to work out.

Cryonics, envisioned in Robert Ettinger's 1962 book *The Prospect of Immortality*, is theoretically based on real science: human embryos are routinely frozen in a process called vitrification, where temperatures below -120 degrees Celsius ensure ice crystals don't form. That's important, because ice crystals tend to destroy cells. This technique preserves biological structure, allowing the embryos to be thawed years later. Their life can literally be paused and then restarted.

The problem with cryonics is that it assumes vitrification of an entire organ, like the brain, or an entire human body, will work as well as when we vitrify a tiny embryo. Cryonics relies on anecdotes of people who survived cold-water immersion or avalanche burials as evidence that rewarming a cold "dead" body can work. But beyond offering suspension of life by freezing, the subsequent rewarming and reanimation part of cryonics remains far-fetched; no one has ever been reanimated after being cryogenically frozen.

The largest organization offering cryonic services is a non-profit called Cryonics Institute. Its president, Dennis Kowalski, has reportedly said, "We have a saying in cryonics: being frozen is the second worst thing that can happen to you. There's no guarantee you'll be able to be brought back, but there is a guarantee that if you get buried or cremated, you'll never find out."

The institute's facility in Clinton, Michigan, which welcomed its first, um, client? in 1977, maintains over one hundred patients in "cryostasis." Rows of vertical cylinders in rooms lit with blue LED lights are prominent on its website, which also has a rather amateur video explaining the process. A link to "emergency situations" guides emergency doctors faced with a potential Cryonics Institute client to continue CPR after death is declared while packing the body with ice to rapidly cool it and injecting it with heparin, a quick-acting blood thinner.

It all seems legit on the surface, but the explanation of how they rapidly cool you falls apart when they talk about a rapid-response team meeting your body at a funeral home to chill it before flying it to Michigan to put it in a liquid nitrogen bath—something I can't see happening within the minutes you have before cellular brain damage begins and starts to erase your memory, personality, and personhood. I suppose the damage might be repairable by future nanotechnology, but it all seems like a stretch to me.

Many have argued against cryonics: if we were to unthaw medieval bodies in the present, concerns about releasing ancient plagues would abound; legal questions around property might surface; and dropping someone into a future world, with cultural, linguistic, and scientific differences, presents moral problems of its own, just as Austin Powers discovered when his sexual advances were rejected and his dental health questioned by his modern counterpart.

While the theoretical arguments around cryonics continue, scientific arguments place cryonics close to science fiction. Vague promises of cell-healing nanobots and neuron-repairing "connectomics" have yet to be shown viable, and suggestions that a person's brain could somehow be mapped into a computer — personality, memories, and all — are nothing short of Star Trek–level postulations. Our best try to date has been in mapping the entire neuroanatomy of the roundworm *Caenorhabditis elegans*, a tiny nematode with 302 neurons. But knowing the synapses that connect these neurons gets us no nearer to uploading a worm brain to a computer.

It's not unreasonable to wonder if cryonics might play a role in modern medicine, but for now, it is merely an aspiration to one day break the circle of life — the prospect of which has inspired hundreds of people to pay hundreds of thousands of dollars each. Still, it raises a question: If cryonically frozen brains are indeed in suspended animation, are they dead at all? The cryonics folks would say no: while you may be legally dead or clinically dead, cryonics defines death as "information-theoretic" death, where the synapses of the brain, where personhood lies, are lost forever. Suspiciously, I was deep into writing this book before I came across the information-theoretic definition of death, which seems restricted to websites promoting cryonics.

Even if you could upload my future brain into a computer, what type of existence would that be? At best, I would live in a world not unlike Keanu Reeves in *The Matrix*, which I suppose would be fun, if not entirely meaningful. But one thing would be true: if the loss of personhood marks the finish line for life, an uploaded brain may very well have succeeded at cheating death.

Brain Transplantation: The Ultimate Technology?

When Sonny Dhanani, the organ transplant expert, and I were chatting, I asked him if we'd see brain transplantation become a reality in the next hundred years. He paused and looked away pensively. "No," he said firmly.

But is the idea that you could transplant my mind into something less fragile and time-bound than a human body, or maybe just into a different human body not consumed with disease, really so far-fetched? Aside from cryogenically freezing my remains in hopes of a future discovery, can we imagine a world where what makes us isn't bound to earthly annoyances like heart failure and kidney disease?

Bear with me here. Let's say a mobster, in a sad case of mistaken identity, shoots you in the head to settle a score. Let's say I have a body riddled with metastatic cancer that has, for now, stayed below the neck. And let's say that doctors put my brain in your body. This is the type of stuff that could one day happen, just as Barnard's heart transplant was a medical marvel back in 1967. (For our purposes here, we'll put aside any discussion of the confusion around who could claim to be the donor and who would be the recipient, not to mention the fact that I would look and maybe even sound like you.)

First, we have to differentiate head transplantation from brain transplantation.

A neurosurgeon once grafted the head of a rhesus monkey onto the body of another rhesus monkey. While the spinal cord wasn't functional and the monkey couldn't move, both body and brain lived eight days before immunorejection got in the way and killed off the amalgamated beast. That was back in 1970. Before it died, the monkey bit the hand of the researcher, so it must have had some sense left in it. Other experiments with dogs ended similarly: the body was able to provide blood flow to the brain, but the brain was unable to provide instructions to the body. They were, in essence, two organisms in series. Yet still, in 2017, Italian surgeons swapped heads on two human corpses, and a 2019 article in the Greek medical journal *Maedica* proposed a surgical technique for head transplantation, showing it's still on the mind of neurosurgeons.

Now, back to brain transplantation. Most scientists will agree that it's impossible to splice the top bit of the spinal cord that exits the brain with another spinal cord that serves the body. Spinal cord injury causing paralysis continues to be an unsolved medical disaster, with wheelchair-bound paraplegic and quadriplegic people affected for the rest of their lives.

But brain transplantation may not necessarily require transplanting the entire brain and splicing together the spinal cord. The brain, in addition to being split into two hemispheres, has an "upstairs" and a "downstairs," and personhood resides in the upstairs. Could this upper part of the brain, the cortex, be detached and implanted onto someone else's downstairs, the cerebellum?

Any possibility of such a procedure being successful is entirely theoretical, and a bad theory at that. Taking one human's brain and inserting it into another human's body isn't going to happen anytime soon; brain transplantation as a way to escape death is as nonviable as reanimating a cryogenically frozen person. For now, anyway.

So, if not transplanting my brain into someone, or something, else, what about uploading it, creating a digitized me? What about cyborgs?

Science fiction has long proposed the idea of human minds being uploaded into robots, computers, and alternate universes. What if, through scientific advancement, this were possible? Could you exist in computer code, lines of ones and zeros?

The scientific term for uploading the human mind

is "whole brain emulation," and the result would be a computer that generates output resembling a sentient, conscious mind—a life-extension technology if ever there was one.

Kenneth Miller, a professor of neuroscience at Columbia University, doesn't think it will happen. In his writings, he describes the complexity of the task. The brain is far too dynamic, with constantly occurring electrical and biochemical signals between neurons. Taking a snapshot of the brain is virtually impossible for at least a few hundred years. But never say never.

A close runner up to the cyborg is artificial intelligence created as a mirror image of a particular person. This gets really creepy, but essentially researchers believe it's possible to create an AI program that is "neuromorphic"—inspired by a particular human brain. In other words, you could create an AI robot and program it to match to a person's personality characteristics.

So while the science that allows organs to be switched from one human to another has advanced dramatically in recent years, doctors still haven't sorted out how to transfer one's personhood to another body or machine.

But let's say, hypothetically, that was possible. What's the result? Let's say my brain is transplanted into your body. My ideas are spoken with your voice. My emotions speak through your eyes. My personality expressed on your face. And my nervous system powering your body to do as I please. What is that result? Is this person me? You? Something new?

While it's fascinating to contemplate, there remains no getting away from the fact that, yes, we do all have to die.

(Sorry, Professor Steiner. I flipped it upside down, but the idea of immortality fell flat.)

CHAPTER 10

Mors Vincit Omnia —
Death Conquers All

IT MIGHT NOT SURPRISE you to hear that other ICU doctors have written books about the death dilemma. Far senior to me, those doctors have summarized medical science, reinforced ethical foundations, and postulated about how to bring a dignified death to the masses. I've read every one of these books and still was left with the grave discomfort I've laid out in these pages.

One of the first books on this topic, aside from Margaret Lock's seminal work *Twice Dead*, was written twenty years before I began writing mine. *Managing Death in the ICU: The Transition from Cure to Comfort*, edited by Randall Curtis and Gordon Rubenfeld, describes the limitations of technology (and there was far less of it in 2001, when the book was published) and shares how to communicate with families the realities of those medical limitations. It also shares

254 • ACCEPTING DEATH AS A PART OF LIFE

with doctors how to ensure comfort at the end of life.

When I first came across *Managing Death*, I felt it would be the holy grail, the answer to my problems. But in its well-referenced and thoughtful pages, I found it ran up against the same problems that I face now, gave the same communication tips that fail me now, and the tension it identified between families and ICU professionals seems worse now than ever.

About a year after I read *Managing Death*, one of its two editors, both of whom are giants in the field, was giving a grand rounds lecture that Stanford was part of. Randall Curtis, professor of palliative and critical care medicine at Harborview Medical Center at the University of Washington, was coming live to a Zoom call, and I had to ask him about the death dilemma.

Little did I know that his talk would lead me to rewrite the last chapter of my own book. Dr. Curtis had recently been diagnosed with ALS — a progressive neuromuscular disease that is fatal about three to five years after symptoms begin — something I hadn't previously been aware of, and at the end of his presentation, tearful colleagues praised his lifetime of dedication to their profession. It was remarkably touching, and lost in the significance of his diagnosis, I didn't ask any questions.

I decided instead to email him. He replied the next day, signing off "Randy."

"I'm being careful with my speaking time these days because of the ALS," he told me, and he asked that we continue to email back and forth instead of talking. We corresponded over the month of June, digging deep into the unsolved matters in our books, gaps that, despite his efforts and those of many others, hadn't been closed.

Randy wrote that much has changed in the twenty years since his book was published. In his eyes, compared to 2001, not as much time and energy is spent convincing ICU doctors of the importance of supporting family members and offering palliative care. "The biggest challenge," he wrote, "is to consistently implement best practices around palliative care and communication about prognosis and shared decision-making." The rub, he elaborated, was in the prognosis: How could we differentiate false hope from true hope?

"The unfortunate reality is that our ability to prognosticate about survival and future quality of life are inherently limited and will always create a tension that needs to be addressed incorporating uncertainty." Emphasizing that emotional support for patients and families can help them prepare for their role in shared decision-making, Randy also added that physicians must do more and be more willing to "bear the burden involved in helping with shared decision-making."

"We trained a generation of physicians," he told me, "who were so steeped in the principle of 'patient autonomy' and the fallibility of prognostication, that many doctors abandon patients and their families to this difficult decision-making without a willingness to truly participate. Obviously, autonomy is very important and our ability to prognosticate is inherently limited, but using these two issues as a shield to avoid fully engaging in the difficult process of helping and supporting patients and their families through difficult decision-making does a disservice to them."

I thought I knew what he was getting at: the decision to withdraw life support or limit technological therapies is a hard one, and one that some families just aren't willing to take responsibility for. Yet those same families say things like "He wouldn't want this" or "She was ready to die." They equivocate, and many physicians turn a blind eye and fail to read between the lines.

I asked Randy to be more explicit. "Some family members want us to take responsibility for these decisions and—in the right circumstances—we should be willing to do that," he wrote.

He shared an anecdote. "When I was a young ICU attending, I took care of an elderly man who had been in a MVC [motor vehicle collision] suffering many injuries and went on to develop multiple organ failure. It was clear to me that though he might survive, he would likely need permanent nursing home placement. His wife was clear that he wouldn't want ongoing life support in these circumstances, but she could not bring herself to make that decision. They had been married many years, and she had been driving the car when the MVC occurred. I remember very clearly her telling me he wouldn't want to continue like this, but she simply couldn't make that decision. The intensivists before me had interpreted that as meaning that life support should continue. I told her, 'You don't have to make that decision. Your job is to tell me what you think your husband would want. My job is to make the decision that your husband would want me to make.' She looked at me with a huge expression of relief and said, 'You can do that?' She was incredibly grateful that I was willing to bear the responsibility of that decision."

Reading this, a lightbulb went off in my head. I wanted to scream "Yes!" This was the missing piece of the puzzle! In the ICU, the doctors knew the dismal prognosis, and so did the family, but neither was willing to make the difficult call to lessen, not maximize, the use of technology that would, in all likelihood, only temporarily postpone death. Could I simply make the interpretation on behalf of my patients, based on what their families could tell me, and propose ending the use of technology?

Randy reminded me that doctors and families both have to be on the side of what the patient would have wanted. "Many family members will not let the physician make that decision and, clouding the difference between what they would want and what the patient would want, fall back to uncertainty about what the patient would want." If the family cannot present a clear picture of the patient's own values and wishes, the doctors cannot implement those values and wishes.

"Nonetheless," he added, "being willing and able to bear the burden of this responsibility — when the circumstances are right — is very important!"

Having finally had a revelation about how I, in my own role as an ICU doctor, can help families and patients address the technology that surrounds them, I decided to ask Randy about how his own disease had impacted his thoughts on dying in an icu.

"My experience has underscored the importance of focusing on the patient's values and goals, rather than on the specific treatments. For me, a PEG [a tube placed through the abdominal wall into the stomach to allow feeding when swallowing is impaired] is a perfect example. I think many critical care clinicians think there is no way they would want a PEG. I would never want a PEG for progressive dementia, but for ALS—it depends."

Randy has what is known as bulbar ALS, which means he will lose his oropharyngeal muscle control—his speech and ability to swallow—before his limbs and respiratory muscles weaken. "It is entirely possible that I will be considering a PEG while I'm still running five miles a day!" he said.

In our email exchanges, I had achieved so much clarity and insight into my role in the death dilemma. And Randy made sure to give me an additional caution, which I found humbling: "Take very seriously the responsibility and obligations that come with prognostication. I think young physicians often have too much or too little confidence in their ability to prognosticate. Experience is a very important part of prognostication. Be very thoughtful and self-reflective about what your prognostication is based on for each patient and to confirm your prognosis with others—other physicians, nurses.... Be sure that your prognostication is not influenced by your personal values around an acceptable quality of life."

With that, I felt, I could write, or rather rewrite, the final chapter of this book.

IT WAS OCTOBER, WHICH is the best month to be a flight paramedic. The leaves in Ontario were changing, and if you were flying further north, you could watch the forests three thousand feet below you go from green to yellow to orange to red. It's one of the most beautiful sights. But this time we were headed south, across Lake Ontario from Billy Bishop Toronto City Airport to the Niagara Falls region, and below us was nothing but blue. A woman had been struck by a dump truck, and I was expecting we'd get called off by the ambulance crew on the ground as soon as they arrived; when a dump truck hits you, Policy 4.4 often comes into full effect.

To my surprise, the cancellation never came. Instead, the crew on scene asked us to re-route to nearby St. Catharines General Hospital as they were already in full "load and go" mode with the patient and we were still ten minutes away. Our pilots vectored us thirty degrees west, and a few minutes later, we touched down on the pad.

Inside the community hospital, Bernie, an emergency doctor I had worked with previously, was placing chest tubes — plastic chutes about the size of those big straws you drink bubble tea with — into the patient's chest. Blood spilled out onto the floor. The paramedics recounted their work: they had, for a few seconds, felt a pulse, which returned for even fewer seconds after some rounds of CPR and an injection of epinephrine.

Bernie had already called for blood from the transfusion lab, and the hospital's on-call surgeon was heading in to see the injured woman. Her blood pressure was critically low — 60 — and she lost her pulse on and off while we poured blood into her veins only to see it come out of her chest tubes.

You're almost never too sick to get into my helicopter — trauma patients have the best chance of survival when we get them to a trauma centre with a trauma surgeon and trauma nurses — but this woman was so unstable, we decided to keep her where she was and resuscitate her with blood. The local surgeon drove in from home while we were working on her, took one look at the patient and went pale. He refused to take a woman so broken to the operating room, which was reasonable, because he hadn't operated in someone's chest for over a decade. (In many community hospitals, general surgeons stick to working in the abdominal cavity to remove gall bladders, bits of bowel, and chunks of cancer, amongst other things.)

After about an hour, we felt we could try a Hail Mary flight to the trauma hospital. The patient's hemoglobin level had stabilized, the pH was now 6.89, up from "undetectable," and we were giving blood, vasopressors, and bicarbonate to keep her alive. It was a fifteen-minute flight to Hamilton General, where I was doing my emergency residency at the time, and so we made a run for it. As soon as the helicopter spooled up, the patient's pulse became faint, then went absent. We took turns doing CPR and squeezing bags of blood into her while alarms pierced through the sound of the engines six inches above our head. I radioed to Hamilton to have help ready on the roof for us.

We landed and immediately unloaded, the wash from the rotors seemingly rushing us along. We went down eight floors in the elevator to get to the ER and sped down the back hall towards Trauma 4. There, about ten people were waiting, including Paul Engels, a trauma team leader who I desperately tried to emulate and hoped to be like one day.

I began spewing the story, rhyming off everything Bernie and I had done, reciting the transfusion count: fourteen red cell bags, eight frozen plasma, all the platelets St. Catharines had, which was two units. Engels wasn't listening. He placed an ultrasound probe on the patient, looked at the screen, and said, "Stop. We're done."

And then he walked away.

At the time, I was incredibly angry. How, after nearly an hour and a half of resuscitation, of throwing the kitchen sink at this lady to get her to the trauma centre, were we done?

Now, as I wrap up my investigation into the death dilemma, I see that Dr. Engels had seen the big picture. I was tunnel-visioned on the pH, on the chest tubes, on the transfusions, but the big picture was clear: this woman had devastating injuries to her chest, to her head, to her abdomen, to her limbs. To anyone standing six feet back, it was very clear: the dump truck had won.

And in this realization, I can see that in my own work now in the ICU, where I work so hard to save each life, I still become tunnel-visioned. I don't want to give up. I stare at computer screens and see lab values change, see urine bags fill, see ECG blips, and I interpret my care as being effective. I'm in adrenalin-pumping resuscitate mode, and it's hard to get out of it, to step back and ask, "Is this really working? Where are we going with this? Is it time to flip the plan and palliate?"

For doctors, it's so hard. Palliative care specialists like Nadia Tremonti and Chris Blake know that. They want to help us see that the light at the end of tunnel can be different from what we expected. Those of us charged with saving lives must also commit to stepping back and re-evaluating our goals, the patient's goals. When we do, we might be like that ICU doctor in medical school who nearly broke my spirit when he kept flipping the plan—and that's not only okay, it's right. As the tunnel towards life is getting longer and longer, the tunnel towards death is getting shorter, its terminal light brighter and brighter. It might not be the tunnel we had hoped to be travelling down, but there is still light at its end, and it's my job to help you see it.

IT'S UNFAIR FOR ME to place blame for the death dilemma solely at the feet of physicians. Often we do what we do because families and patients want us to keep going, even when we're convinced that pursuing further care is wrong. But families have to be part of the solution; they too must pause and reflect, see things as they are, not as they were, just as Steve Berry, the death historian, said people did decades ago, before the luxury of technology. The sunk costs of weeks of visits, meetings, and hoping for a miracle often need to be set aside, and a dispassionate re-evaluation triggered. After one hundred days in the ICU, ask the tough questions: What are the odds of getting out of the ICU? What complications might occur if we continue? The power is in your hands as much as it's in mine.

Who holds the balance of power in weighing the decision to flip the plan depends on where you live. Mike Christian, the Canadian expat living in London, told me that the power balance in the U.K. hasn't shifted towards families the way it has in Canada or the United States.

"There is much more physician autonomy in the U.K. There is less burden placed on families, because the physicians have made this decision, and I think there is some benefit to that.

"In Canada and the U.S., we put a lot of the weight of these decisions on families. I think a lot of doctors take too much of the weight off their shoulders and say, 'It's all the family's decision.' But I find that perplexing. Doctors aren't allowed to treat their own families specifically because we recognize the inability to make good decisions when we are in emotional situations. But then we turn to family members in the ICU and expect them to make these decisions without a medical degree, without the experience you have seeing all these cases over your career. It's really contradictory."

When I ask a family how far they want me to go in treating their loved one, the natural question for them to pose is one of statistics. Everyone wants a number: What are the odds they'll make it? To be honest, with few exceptions, I just guess, and so does Mike. It really doesn't matter if it's 1 percent, 5 percent, or 50 percent, because unless I say "0 percent," families want "everything done"—just like Jafar, the frozen student, would have wanted.

The problem with statistics is that one assumes that if you don't die, you live. Say there is a 5 percent chance of surviving. In ICU speak, that means being able to walk and talk and feed yourself. That doesn't mean there is a 95 percent chance of death. Maybe that's only 60 percent or 70 percent. The other 25 to 35 percent? What many of us would consider a fate worse than death. Life in an LTACH or nursing home or some other existence far from what you knew in healthier times, without the independence that so many of us consider vital to a good life.

I asked Mike if it was realistic to think I could help families manage these impossible decisions by working on my communications skills. But Mike figured I was already a good communicator, just like he was, just like most of us in critical care units are.

"We really need to help the families cope and arrive at the place they need to be, but there are some things you can't change. You are asking someone to think not about themselves but the other person, and the ability for humans to do that varies greatly, and that process doesn't start the day their loved ones become ill or injured. It's developed over their whole life, so expecting to change that is like expecting a miracle. You can't change their personality."

So we have created this situation ourselves in society with the way laws and medicine have evolved, and it clearly hasn't kept up with the way technology has evolved.

"Trying to find the right balance is hard," Mike told me.

Tell me about it.

SOMETIMES, FAMILIES COME TO the table ready to make tough calls.

As I was finishing this book, I admitted a patient who had suffered a fairly significant hemorrhagic stroke while out for a walk. He was elderly and had no identification on him, and the electronic medical record had autogenerated an ID for him: Twenty-five Eighty, 119M.

He of course was not 119 years old, but that's what the computer used as a placeholder.

He was intubated and hooked up to a ventilator and was started on drips to manage his blood pressure. Eventually, the police identified him and brought his wife, who spoke only Mandarin, to visit him. I met her in the ICU room, and we stood over her doomed husband of sixty-five years.

Speaking through a translator on speakerphone, I began to explain how grave the situation was. I felt ready to be definitive, to be explicit, to be hopeless. I did not want this man to end up with a tracheostomy and feeding tube and shipped off to an LTACH. I was going to keep him from falling afoul of the death dilemma, right now, before any other doctors could arrive and paint a rosier picture.

But I didn't have to say much.

The woman immediately said that her husband lived a long life, an independent life, and would never want any machine to keep him alive.

I explained the options we had, and with equal parts sadness and conviction, she asked me to remove the breathing tube.

Through my mask, I smiled at her and she smiled at me. I was relieved. In a flash, the deal was made and she turned to her husband and began rubbing his feet. There was something beautiful about this little old woman rubbing the feet of her unconscious husband. Something tender and committed and heart warming.

She didn't stop until after the respiratory therapist had removed the endotracheal tube and the heart tracing went flat. She looked at me, and I nodded once. She thanked me in Mandarin, then walked out of the room and down the hallway, her heart broken but her mind at ease. She had fulfilled her final duty as his wife, and she was at peace. So was Twenty-five Eighty.

So was I. It was one of those beautiful deaths Chris

Blake made seem so ordinary in his line of work doing palliative care.

It was the death I would want for myself.

IT'S HARD FOR ME to ask you to contemplate your death as you read this book; few people think about their own end until it's thrust upon them by a cancer diagnosis or heart attack or loss of a loved one. So it's not surprising that most ICU patients show up rather unexpectedly, with no documented wishes and having had remarkably few conversations with anyone about how they want to die. But the reality is that, because of technology and medical science, it will become more and more common that doctors are left unable to liberate people from the confines of their hospital bed and present them with a choice: live out their days supported by machines until they die of a complication, or make the decision to turn off the machines and die in peace.

When I first met Jerry, he was trying to escape his hospital bed. Pissed off and combative, he had been in hospital for a few days when he decided he'd had enough and wanted to leave. Tattooed, overweight, and sporting a bushy moustache, he looked like the type of dude who rides his Harley motorcycle from truck stop to truck stop whistling at women along the way.

Jerry's wife and children couldn't convince him to stay for treatment, nor did the veteran charge nurse (also an actual war veteran), who could convince anyone of anything, have any luck. So I got called, the medical student covering internal medicine wards that night.

Jerry would have scared most medical students, but I had seen enough of his type on the road as a medic. I went to the desk and reviewed his chart. Hamilton General hadn't (and still hasn't) implemented electronic records, so his chart was a real chart. (For my contemporary colleagues, it was a three-ring binder with sheets of paper that had ink on them.)

Jerry had diabetes, high blood pressure, and high cholesterol. A combination of those diseases had left his arteries damaged to the point that blood couldn't flow to his feet. This left him with an ulcer on his heel that would be the envy of Hollywood moulage artists preparing extras for a zombie apocalypse movie.

The wound was so bad, bacteria and fungi had snuck deep into it, invading his bloodstream and attaching themselves to his heart valves: infective endocarditis. He essentially had a mushroom growing on his tricuspid valve, and it was affecting the *lub-dub* opening and closing of the valve with each heartbeat. Jerry felt perfectly fine, but it was only a matter of time before the valve failed and the ventricle would pump blood backwards into the atrium. That's bad: blood should only ever flow forward.

Jerry needed to be on IV antifungal and antibiotic drugs for a few days before going to the operating room to have his valve replaced. But he didn't want to wait. He didn't even want to have surgery. He also didn't want to die. Jerry didn't really know what he wanted, and it was now my job to find out.

Years as a paramedic had helped me develop various voices to use in different circumstances: soft and sweet with Granny at the nursing home, calm yet firm with entitled patients spewing demands, strict and forceful with belligerent drunks. Calling on a strange combination of experience, intuition, and theatre skills, I modulated my voice the moment I saw him.

My voice, strong, clear and slightly pissed off, laid out the bottom line for Jerry. I gave him two options: go home and die, or stay in hospital and live. He chose the latter, agreeing to wait, chill out, and be kind to my nurses. (Since he had made the deal with me, I used the term "my nurses" to imply that our deal extended to them.)

The overnight crisis averted, I returned to the litany of other fires that needed extinguishing by the overnight skeleton crew. Jerry would go on to finish his antibiotic course and receive a new heart valve, and the only way I know that is because the cardiovascular ICU called me a few months later while I was on vacation in Southeast Asia.

On a boat in the middle of the Indian Ocean, after a few days of a strict powered-down vacation, I gave in and turned my phone off airplane mode and logged into the satellite Wi-Fi. There was an email from the intensivist, and I opened it.

"Are you around? You saw a guy named Jerry a few months ago, and he's requesting you to come and discontinue his life support."

I read on. Apparently the fungus in Jerry's blood had

gotten into his breastbone, which the surgeons had to
cut in half lengthwise to get access to his heart for the
valve replacement surgery. That was over a month ago.
Jerry had been languishing on a ventilator in the ICU
while the infectious disease doctors tried a litany of
drugs to heal the wound. The surgeons had debrided it.
The intensivists had tried to improve blood flow to it.
But nothing worked. The team had no more tricks up
their sleeves. And Jerry had, once again, had enough.

Jerry had thought my interaction with him way back
that night on the medicine ward was one of the more
honest ones he'd had at the hospital, his wife would
later tell me, and he wanted my opinion about what he
should do. I wasn't able to give him that opinion, being
on the other side of the world at the time, but if I were at
work, I most certainly would have. Ultimately, he asked
that the ventilator be turned off. He received palliative
care and died with his wife at his side.

We don't often see patients make this choice in the
ICU. But I think Jerry's decision was the right one for
him.

LET'S SUMMARIZE. THERE ARE three major players in
the death dilemma, and none of them are ventilators
or ECMO circuits or defibrillators. The first is you, the
patient, who through acts of omission have ended up in
an ICU without a plan of your own, without clear wishes
guiding your care. The second is your family, who,
grief-stricken and hopeful, are running blind, asked by

doctors to arrive at choices that sound impossible to make. At best, they are guessing what you would want them to do; at worst, they are so consumed with their own emotions they aren't making any decisions at all. And third, there is me. Along with my colleagues in nursing, respiratory care, pharmacy, hematology, nutrition, and with countless other folks employed by the institution to stare at numbers on computer screens, we set out to save your life, and get so wrapped up in the minutiae that we can forget to step back and see the forest through the trees.

Each of these three players has the power to end the death dilemma by exercising their judgement when it comes to applying technology to the dying process, and more times than not, compassionate and caring people can come to the right decision for each patient and death comes at the right time, in the right way. How do we increase the good deaths, then, and reduce the bad? Let's revisit the death dilemma equation:

$$Technology$$
$$\times$$
$$(Resuscitation\ Glorification + Death\ Denialism)$$
$$=$$
$$False\ Hope$$

To solve the equation, we must first move technology out of its current power-grabbing position and instead consider its use when ethical — and by ethical, I mean not only to prevent immediate death but to reasonably

272 • ACCEPTING DEATH AS A PART OF LIFE

promote a return to life. Just as surgeons can decline
to operate on patients who are unlikely to benefit from
going under the knife, so too must ER and ICU doctors
draw clear lines when faced with dismal prospects. Preventing immediate death is not, in itself, a valid enough
reason to apply lifesaving technology. Of course, there
will be times when the prognosis is unclear and the
patient's values are unclear — out comes the kitchen
sink, to buy us time. But this choice to initiate life support must be revisited; initiating and sustaining tech
are two different ball games.

The decision to initiate technological life support can
be elucidated by an understanding of the prognosis and
of the values of the patient. Before accepting technological life support, patients and their families must be
fully informed of their choices. This is the major failure
of the status quo: doctors provide scripted spiels seeking
informed consent for procedures like tracheostomy or
ECMO cannulation while withholding the truth about
the long road to recovery patients will face, the likelihood of painful complications, and the alternatives to
these actions, primarily palliative care. The "need" for
technology, as often presented by physicians, is cloaked
in resuscitation glorification and death denialism, and
without more information of the real cost of pursuing resuscitation, and blind to the values of palliation,
patients and their families are often left with an impression that there is no choice but to accept technology.

The use of technology, if it's chosen to be applied at
all, must be frequently reassessed with grace, humility,

and the patient's preferences foremost in mind, and with a full understanding of all therapeutic options — technological, medical and palliative. Families must be guided away from resuscitation glorification with the help of doctors who inform them about what any long road to recovery might entail, who provide them with realistic estimates of the impact technology will have, and are better at breaking down what the outcomes will look like so they and the patient themselves can decide what course of action is acceptable.

It is too common for doctors to sugar-coat the pill by saying things like "nothing is getting worse" or "the white cell count is going down" or "the chest X-ray is improved," micro-improvements that may mean nothing in the grand scheme of things. While seemingly benign, these encouraging comments strengthen death denialism by creating a fallacy that the patient is inching closer to recovery. Death denialism can also be addressed by entertaining dual priorities, pursuing both aggressive resuscitation while still discussing early on the availability of palliative measures and potential junctures at which to introduce them. Without knowing what this flipping of the plan to palliation might look like, or at what point it would be in accordance with the patient's values, families are left with no alternative but to push forward with aggressive, potentially futile care that increases suffering.

Should it be deemed that the risk of suffering is greater than the risk of acceptable recovery — and I mean acceptable to the patient, not the surgeon or physician caring for the patient—then palliative care should be invoked. Both the ethical application of technology and the weighting of risk and benefit of ongoing care are best served when these two factors have been contemplated by individuals ahead of acute illness, and discussed with their loving family members such that they are understood and accepted. Certainly, having an advance directive that lays out limits of care makes everyone's job easier and less distressing.

Of course, doctors like me must stay humble, recognizing the challenges of prognostication, especially early on in critical illness. I would hate for this book to embolden doctors to give up too early on patients, before the impact of technology is truly known, when families might be a little too trusting of us when we say, with good intentions but less-than-good accuracy, that "this won't end well." The death dilemma, in many cases, shouldn't factor into the initial resuscitation, or the first few days in the ICU, unless the clinical condition, or the patient's wishes, are exceptionally clear.

When relationships between the three stakeholders in the death dilemma become acrimonious, all three lose control, and the situation becomes intractable. The status quo is set up to respond to these breakdowns by extending decision-making to other players instead. Courts are left to decide, a seemingly reasonable but pragmatically disastrous process that takes years to sort out. Ethicists have to make unilateral decisions, generating headlines in newspapers and sadness on all sides of the debate. We can leave it to God, deferring decisions that humans were gifted the ability to make on their own and ignoring the loss of grace, dignity, and peace. We can leave it to science, in which case us doctors can keep a person in the grey zone seemingly indefinitely as we watch in horror their skin breaking down and muscle wasting away until no one can recognize anymore who we are trying to help. Agony and financial bankruptcy seem to be the only two outcomes in this max-out-the-science approach.

I know we can all do better. I know we can conquer the death dilemma. The solution lies within us, and it's a capacity that, time and time again, humans have demonstrated they possess. I can prove it, with the story of a rhinoceros named Sudan.

NAJIN AND HER DAUGHTER, Fatu, are the last two northern white rhinoceroses on earth. Despite being healthy, the rhinos, second only to elephants as the largest land mammals on earth, are already functionally extinct. Najin's father, Sudan, was the last male of the subspecies to grace East Africa. When he died, on March 19, 2018, Najin and Fatu were fated to become emblems of the past. Once numbering in the thousands, the wild population of the northern white rhino was wiped out by civil war and poaching; their horns, gram for gram, are worth more than gold.

Sudan had been a celebrity in Kenya. Tourists flocked to see him at the Ol Pejeta Conservancy, where armed guards protected him twenty-four hours a day and scientists committed thousands of hours to studying him. After his death, he became a global sensation, with features in the *New York Times* and *National Geographic*, and in news broadcasts around the world.

At forty-five years old, it was well known Sudan's days were numbered. Weeks before he died, he was slowing down, becoming weak. He had wounds that would not heal despite the efforts of the veterinarians. His sperm was frozen in a San Diego laboratory so that northern white rhinos could perhaps enjoy a Jurassic Park–style comeback in the future, but everyone at Ol Pejeta was growing sombre as reality crept up on them.

The day Sudan died, he was surrounded by the keepers who'd fought so hard over the past decades for the northern white rhino to survive. Sudan had lain down just before sunset the night before and was now too weak to stand. He was fed bananas with pain pills mushed inside. His keepers talked to him. He was caressed. He was loved. And then, fully aware that they were wiping a magnificent mammal off the face of the planet, they euthanized him. Their devastation was captured in photos that went viral worldwide.

If the caretakers who loved him so much could bring themselves to help Sudan towards death, bringing functional extinction to the northern white rhinoceros in the process, then surely we can recognize the rightful end of a human life too and allow our own loved ones to die a dignified death unencumbered by machines.

ASSUMING TECHNOLOGY WILL ONLY become more imposing, and that people in our society will continue to resist contemplating their own demise, leaving them without a plan when they unexpectedly end up in the ICU, doctors like me will continue to battle families.

How do we get to the same page, to the same shared principles of humanism, love, and death acceptance? That is essentially the question I have been trying to answer since I started writing this book.

The palliative care folks who peddle communications workshops and the psychologists who select phrases to get through to people are well intentioned. They are academic and thorough in their efforts. But their efforts are half measures, Band-Aids that cover a deeper divide between doctors and the patients and families who wind up in the ICU, where perhaps more than anywhere else in the hospital, the patients are sickest, tensions are highest, and time is shortest.

This sets up a communication disaster: doctors have time only to blurt out facts, and families have no chance to explore their fears and values.

What's worse, the training doctors receive from palliative care specialists and psychologists can leave us with the impression we can win the difficult conversations, that we can pull a manoeuvre to get what we want. This us-versus-them approach, the framing of end-of-life conversations as a debate, sets us up to fail.

In his book *Think Again: The Power of Knowing What You Don't Know*, organizational behaviour expert

Adam Grant, a Wharton School professor, uses a term that struck me hard.

"Logic bully."

Logic bullies focus on what *they* know, using facts as weapons to change people's minds. But once a mind is made up, facts tend not to change your stance. Their opponent, firmly of an opposite opinion, begins to selectively refute those facts with facts or beliefs of their own. The two sides dig in, and we get nowhere.

I have realized that I am a logic bully. When families disagree with me, I load them up with facts, exerting my expertise on what is presumably a rational decision-making process but which is clearly driven by emotion.

Grant suggests abandoning your inner logic bully in favour of becoming a curious motivational interviewer. In motivational interviewing, the physician tries to call attention to nuances in people's positions. Psychologists find that, with this technique, people become less extreme. By inquiring about someone's position, you can open their mind to change.

Logic bullies seize on "sustain talk," which is about maintaining the status quo, such as marshalling facts or beliefs that buttress a position. But skilled motivational interviewers monitor conversations for "change talk," listening for references to a desire, ability, or commitment to make a shift.

Every medical student is taught some form of motivational interviewing, but only in passing. Although there is plenty of evidence supporting motivational interviewing, such as studies showing it increases willingness to receive vaccination, it remains a hokey exercise for the unpracticed, like when I have to attend workshops on breaking bad news. To do it well requires practice and skill, and for those who become expert at it, it leads to better relationships with patients and their families and opens the door to flipping the plan. But it's not always enough.

As Grant said in a *New York Times* opinion piece, "I no longer believe it's my place to change anyone's mind. All I can do is try to understand their thinking and ask if they're open to some rethinking. The rest is up to them."

It's on doctors like me to really understand people's motivations for wanting an abundance of medical technology even after it's clear to all sides that death is the inevitable outcome. In reflecting on this new model of communication, where we abandon our efforts to score points and come out the winner, doctors can recentre decisions around the patient whose fate depends so literally on these life-and-death discussions.

Simply put, us doctors must set ego aside and inject ourselves with a dose of curiosity. We must learn about our patients' values and beliefs. We must listen to the fears of families. Only then can we start to advocate for our patients using our respect for science but also our love for humanity.

I LEFT MY JOB as a paramedic because I wanted to know what happened next, a gap in my work satisfaction that followed me into the ER. But now in the ICU, I don't feel the same emptiness, the same desire to follow people into the wards, or to rehab, or to their homes. I now understand that when they asked me in my medical school interview at McMaster why I wanted to be a doctor, I was being literal when I said, "To save lives."

It's natural, then, that when I can't save lives, I hunker down, go into denial, and keep trying. Sometimes, I do that with a clear mind and a true belief that I can yet save a life. Other times, it's the path of least resistance, an attempt to assuage my own guilt, or a well-intentioned offering to a grieving family. Oddly, hooking people up to life support is often the easiest thing to do.

But as Ron Stewart knows from his fifty years as a physician, at some point, the role of a doctor is to call it, to say, "We're done here. Nothing good can come from continuing to resuscitate." That sounds easy enough, and I know that palliation, providing a dignified death, is nearly as rewarding as saving a life. But when families don't trust me to know when the moment to call it has arrived, I'm stuck. We all are.

As a physician, I need to earn trust to represent not only the best medical science but also the earnest execution of how to apply that science to the individual patient I am charged with caring for. That means recognizing and communicating with remarkable transparency and honesty the limitations of medical science and realities of the end of life.

Death conquers all, because everything has its limits. Yet in accepting death, we become limitless, freed from the suffering experienced by the immortal Tithonus. Mortality is perhaps the most ubiquitous human trait, one we must not only accept, but embrace. Be it by a faith in the afterlife or a belief in the body's biochemical return to nature, death can be viewed not as the end but as a transition point that must come. If we are to believe in the stories of J. R. R. Tolkien, death comes as a compassionate offering from God.

What can I say in the ICU when tensions are high and emotions catastrophic? I think back to my days as a paramedic and the times when a heart was too sick to beat or lungs too sick to take oxygen, where the simplicity of it all brought clarity to the finality of death. That suddenness had its advantages. In the ICU, death is a process that must be reconciled not just clinically but philosophically too. I'll be doing everything I can to break away from the false dichotomy of "resuscitate or palliate" and merge together the efforts both to save a life and attend to its final hours.

When ICU doctors love their patients and understand their families, and when families understand the limitations of medicine at the end of life, we can form an alliance to honour a person's life with a loving end.

While our communication skills have developed more slowly than medical technology, the death dilemma is not really about doctors pitted against families, a simple translation error between the languages of science and emotion. We all speak a common language, the language of love. And in loving life, we must also find a space in us to desire a death that comes at the right time. A death that is without suffering or pain or anxiety. A death that is comfortable, meaningful, and dare I say, beautiful.

After writing this book, my commitment to saving lives is stronger than ever, but so is my commitment to advocating for a dignified death free of suffering, a death we all are due, not a moment too soon or a moment too late.

Conclusion:
What Should You Do Now That
You've Read This Book?

I'M NOT SURE WHAT made you pick up this book. Perhaps you have a family member or friend who's gravely ill. Perhaps you've been given a troubling diagnosis. Perhaps you were the one to make a call about withdrawing life support or authorizing long-term care and want reassurance you did the right thing. Or perhaps, like me, you find the death dilemma fascinating, a confusing collision of science, religion, law, and society. Regardless, you've come this far, and you probably want to know what to do next.

STEP ONE: Think about death. This is something you've already been doing, so you can move on to step two.

STEP TWO: Talk about death. It's often easiest to do this with your friends first, to make it all make sense and to contextualize what you've read in this book with your own values and beliefs. Then talk to your family. They may not like the idea of one day pulling the plug on Grandma or sending Dad to a nursing home. But have the tough conversations now, when the pressure is off and everyone is calm and rational. Delaying the conversation until it's unavoidable doesn't usually work out so well. (You can trust me on this one.)

STEP THREE: Write about death. Get your wishes down on paper, with legal advice. Make sure the person you designate to carry out your wishes agrees to do so. Make sure your documentation is authentic and complete, or it may not stand up to family infighting when you're not able to speak up for yourself. Consider registering as an organ donor; let something good come of tragedy. And keep these documents up to date; as your life evolves, so too might your thinking on death.

STEP FOUR: Live your life. As an emergency doctor, I am reminded daily that death is inevitable but far from predictable. Live well—it's certainly easier to live your life when you've already planned for your death. I'm not saying you should blow your life savings on a first-class ticket to Australia, but I see so many hard working people lose everything they have built in an instant and miss out on the chance to reap the rewards of their labour. Find a balance between experiencing joy now and saving for later.

When the time comes, perhaps we'll meet in the ICU. I'll commit to doing everything I can to save your life. And if I can't, I'll wish you a good death; not a moment too soon or a moment too late.

Acknowledgements

I MUST EXTEND MY sincere gratitude to a number of people who were instrumental in my journey to write *Death Interrupted*.

First, to my editor, Alex Schultz, for his remarkable ability to read a doctor's handwriting and clarify a doctor's thoughts, and to Douglas Richmond, for his wise guidance producing the book. Second, to Lauren McKeon, who skillfully edited the essay that I eventually expanded to become *Death Interrupted*. To the entire team at House of Anansi Press and The Walrus, for seeing a complex story in need of exploration and for trusting me to tell it.

To my mentors in health care, particularly Randy Wax, Andrew Healey, Alison Fox-Robichaud, Michelle Welsford, Laurie Morrison, Alan Craig, and Rebecca Aslakson, who have helped me process the weight of what we do daily, and taught me how to combine science and humanity into a medical practice.

To my colleagues in the ER and ICU: social workers, nurses, respiratory therapists, dieticians, unit clerks, paramedics, physicians, and learners, who make this work environment emotionally sustainable.

To my Pegasus Writers group, led by Jenn Pien, for their investment in me as a writer and love they have shown to me throughout writing *Death Interrupted*, and my dear friend Chris Blake for his literary insights.

To Gaibrie Stephen, for his excellent reporting on narcotics in Ohio and beyond, and to Rob Steiner, for teaching me how to apply journalistic tradecraft to everything I do. And to Seema Marwaha for her career guidance as I blend medicine and writing.

To my best friends, Thomas, Bob, Siobán, Sumeet, and Sus; the knowledge that you are always there for me allows me to dare and sleep soundly at night.

To my partner Fernando Valencia, whose unconditional encouragement pushed me to delve into dark places to find flickers of light.

My parents deserve credit for raising me to chirp at the norm, a habit that aids me as both a physician and journalist. My sister Heather also deserves thanks for being my partner in crime in our developmental years.

And lastly, but most importantly, to each person who spoke to me about the death dilemma. Your stories enriched *Death Interrupted* and deepened my own understanding of what it means to die, to live, and to be somewhere in between.

Author's Note

There are certain times I was restricted, by professional ethics, from divulging details about a person or place. In those circumstances, I constructed composites that reflect my true experiences over seventeen years caring for critically ill people. I did my best to be descriptive and true without violating the trust people place in me as a doctor, colleague, and friend.

There may be other circumstances where my account of an event is coloured by the stress of emergency care or the passage of time, or where I took liberty with the chronology of events to weave a coherent story. Any errors are unintentional, regrettable, and entirely my responsibility.

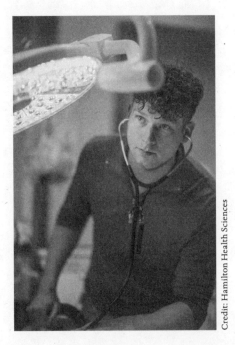

DR. BLAIR BIGHAM is a journalist, scientist, and attending emergency and ICU physician who trained at McMaster and Stanford Universities. He was a Global Journalism Fellow at the Munk School of Global Affairs and an associate scientist at St. Michael's Hospital. His work has appeared in the *Toronto Star*, the *Globe and Mail*, the *New England Journal of Medicine*, and the *Canadian Medical Association Journal*, among others.